The Inside Story on

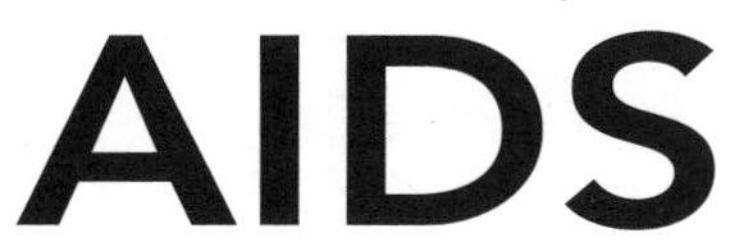

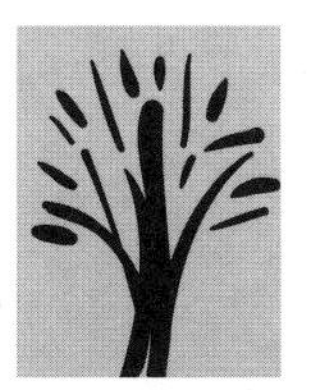

The Inside Story on AIDS

Experts Answer Your Questions

Seth C. Kalichman, PhD

American Psychological Association • Washington, DC

Published by
APA LifeTools
American Psychological Association
750 First Street, NE
Washington, DC 20002
www.apa.org

To order
APA Order Department
P.O. Box 92984
Washington, DC 20090-2984

Tel: (800) 374-2721; Direct: (202) 336-5510
Fax: (202) 336-5502; TDD/TTY: (202) 336-6123
Online: www.apa.org/books/
E-mail: order@apa.org

In the U.K., Europe, Africa, and the Middle East, copies may be ordered from
American Psychological Association
3 Henrietta Street
Covent Garden, London
WC2E 8LU England

Typeset in Minion by World Composition Services, Inc., Sterling, VA

Printer: Automated Graphic Systems, White Plains, MD
Cover Designer: Naylor Design, Washington, DC
Technical/Production Editor: Kristen R. Sullivan

Library of Congress Cataloging-in-Publication Data

Kalichman, Seth C.
The inside story on AIDS / by Seth C. Kalichman.
p. cm.
Includes bibliographical references and index.
ISBN 1-55798-984-2 (alk. paper)
1. AIDS (Disease)—Popular works. 2. AIDS (Disease)—Miscellanea. I. Title.

RC606.64.K35 2003
616.97′92—dc21 2002034188

British Library Cataloguing-in-Publication Data
A CIP record is available from the British Library.

Printed in the United States of America
First Edition

To Moira and Hannah
for answering so many of my questions.

And to all of those affected by AIDS
for their inspiration.

Contents

Acknowledgments

This book would not have been possible without the help of Kari DiFonzo of the AIDS Resource Center of Wisconsin and Bart Loeser of the Houston AIDS Foundation. Along with their teams of dedicated volunteers, Kari and Bart provided me with the questions that form the basis for this book. I thank Tami Payne who transferred over 3,000 questions from AIDS-line phone log sheets to index cards, making the organization of the original text possible. I am indebted to David Rompa, Michael Lisowski, and David G. Ostrow for their help in evaluating questions and developing answers. I am also lucky to have developed the original idea with Ted Baroody and Olin Nettles at the American Psychological Association (APA), whose original contributions remain very much a part of this book. Thanks also to Julia Frank-McNeil, Mary Lynn Skutley, Susan Reynolds, and Linda McCarter of APA

Books for their commitment to this project. I also wish to thank Rita B. Kalichman who provided me with helpful comments on the clarity of questions and answers and encouraged me to complete the book—her never-ending enthusiasm continues to fuel my interest. I also wish to express my appreciation to Syd Kalichman, who inspires the best in me, and to Billy and Debbie for their support.

The Inside Story on
AIDS

Introduction

My ignorance could cost me my life, but I wanted to try and ensure that no one else would become infected with HIV for the same reason. . . . Now God has said to me, "You've got to let the world know that AIDS is about to become an even bigger epidemic, and you're going to have to teach again."
—Earvin "Magic" Johnson, November 18, 1991

The personal and social tragedy of the AIDS crisis touches everyone. For those of you who have not yet personally known someone stricken by this dreadful disease, it seems that it is only a matter of time before you will. For many of you, celebrities are the first to bring AIDS into your life. Actor Rock Hudson, basketball superstar Magic Johnson, actress and comedian Sandie Church, tennis champion Arthur Ashe, activist Elizabeth Glaser, rock star Freddy Mercury, entertainer and songwriter Peter Allen, ballet dancer

Rudolf Nureyev, activist and author Mary Fisher, MTV personality Pedro Zamora, Olympic diving champion Greg Luganis, and film actor Anthony Perkins—these are among the 30 million people in the world who have been infected with human immunodeficiency virus, or HIV, the virus that causes acquired immune deficiency syndrome, or AIDS. More than 800,000 people have been diagnosed with AIDS in the United States, which is over 300,000 more people than in 1995. More than 460,000 Americans have died. AIDS is one of the leading causes of death of young men and women in U.S. cities, claiming more lives than accidents, murders, cancer, or heart disease.[1]

From the very beginning, education has been the first line of defense against AIDS. In the mid-1980s, the U.S. government launched a national AIDS education campaign that was more massive than any other in history and included mailing information brochures to every home. It was hoped that the public would recognize the urgency of the AIDS crisis, stop believing myths about AIDS, and protect themselves from getting the virus. People were told that AIDS is caused by HIV, a deadly virus that is transmitted from person to person through direct contact with blood and other body fluids, almost always by having sex with an

[1]Centers for Disease Control and Prevention. (2002). *HIV/AIDS surveillance report*. Atlanta, GA: Author. (Available online at www.cdc.gov)

infected person without using latex condoms and sharing needles to inject drugs. The news media, popular press, and the personal tragedies of people infected with HIV affirmed this message. Today, most people are aware of AIDS and are familiar with these simple facts.

A little knowledge can, however, raise many questions and promote misconceptions, albeit unintentionally. Although the fundamental AIDS prevention messages are out, people remain misinformed about many important aspects of AIDS:

- How is HIV not transmitted?
- When don't you have to worry about getting AIDS?
- Can sex ever really be safe?
- What does HIV do to the body?
- What is the difference between HIV and AIDS?
- Who is at greatest risk?
- Is there a cure for AIDS?

The U.S. National Health Interview Survey[2] showed that most everyone knows that having sex with a person who has HIV carries great risk for getting AIDS. However, few people know other basic AIDS

[2]Centers for Disease Control and Prevention, National Center for Health Statistics. (1997). *National Health Interview Survey*. Retrieved October 28, 2002, from http://www.cdc.gov/nchs/nhis.htm#1997%20NHIS

facts. The study showed that two thirds of people wrongly believe that a person is likely to get AIDS from kitchen utensils that were used by someone with AIDS and that three out of four people believe that they can get the virus that causes AIDS by a mere kiss on the cheek, when in fact the virus cannot be transmitted in these ways. Misinformation about AIDS leads to unwarranted fears, undue concerns, and prejudices against people living with the disease. Other misinformation puts people at risk for HIV infection, including beliefs that men cannot get HIV from women, that condoms make sex completely safe, and that getting tested for HIV protects people from later getting the virus.

Every day in the United States, hundreds of people dedicate their time to answering questions about AIDS that come through AIDS information hotlines. For example, according to the American Social Health Association, the National AIDS Hotline receives 2,700 calls per day, or about 1 million calls per year! The questions that the American public asks about AIDS form the basis for this book.

My idea of writing this book began when students in my college classes started asking me about the epidemic. I wondered if my students' questions were like those of the general public, so I contacted hotlines in two cities, Milwaukee, Wisconsin, and Houston, Texas. I selected these two cities because they are located in the middle of America. I visited the hotline operators and collected questions asked more recently.

I also searched the Internet for question-and-answer AIDS Web pages. The AIDS-line workers at the AIDS Resource Center of Wisconsin and Houston AIDS Foundation have responded to thousands of questions about AIDS. Professionals and volunteers there helped me by writing down more than 1,600 questions that people have asked. My research with people receiving services at public health clinics confirmed that the very same questions were often asked in clinics. As an AIDS prevention researcher, I also knew that there were answers to all of their questions.

This book represents a collection of questions that people phoned into AIDS hotlines and asked online. This is not the first book written about AIDS, nor will it be the last. But it is one of the first that tries to answer the questions that you may actually have about AIDS—not the questions experts think you have. My approach is that every question is worth asking. This book answers questions with currently available scientific information. People often ask questions that are difficult to answer, questions for which there is incomplete information, questions that leave room for ambiguous answers. Nevertheless, I have included questions that cannot be answered completely at this time, noting the current state of knowledge.

Much of the mistaken information people have comes in the form of half-truths taken to be "The Truth" or taken from news reports of a single research finding. The answers in this book are based on scientific studies. The AIDS epidemic has brought forth its own language, so a glossary of terms is included. Where there is still uncertainty or controversy, I point it out. However, readers should be aware that information about AIDS is rapidly changing. More has been learned about AIDS in a short time than any other disease in history. We know a lot about AIDS, and it is my goal to share this information by answering your questions.

Before reading further, please take a few minutes to complete the following AIDS assessment. This objective test, which was adapted from an HIV knowledge test by Dr. Michael Carey and his colleagues at Syracuse University, includes a wide range of questions about AIDS-related facts. This well-developed and scientifically sound test represents much of what is known about AIDS. You can use it as a self-test to see what gaps you may have in your own knowledge about AIDS. Correct answers to the questions are located in the back of the book (Appendix B), along with other resources for answering your questions about AIDS.

HIV/AIDS Knowledge Questionnaire[3]

Answer each question the best that you can, circling either Yes or No, or DK if you do not know an answer.

1.	HIV and AIDS are the same thing.	T	F	DK
2.	There is a cure for AIDS.	T	F	DK
3.	A person can get AIDS from a toilet seat.	T	F	DK
4.	Coughing and sneezing DO NOT cause HIV.	T	F	DK
5.	A person can get HIV by sharing an injection needle with someone who has HIV.	T	F	DK
6.	A person can get HIV if she or he has sex with someone who has HIV.	T	F	DK
7.	HIV can be spread by mosquitoes.	T	F	DK
8.	AIDS is the cause of HIV.	T	F	DK
9.	A person can get HIV by sharing a glass of water with someone who has HIV.	T	F	DK
10.	A person can get HIV by shaking hands with someone who has HIV.	T	F	DK
11.	HIV is killed by bleach.	T	F	DK
12.	It is possible to get HIV when a person gets a tattoo.	T	F	DK

[3]*Note*. From *HIV Knowledge Questionnaire*, by M. P. Carey, 1997, Syracuse, NY: Syracuse University. Used with permission.

13. A man can get HIV if he has sex with another man who has HIV. T F DK
14. A pregnant woman with HIV can give the virus to her unborn baby. T F DK
15. Pulling out the penis before a man climaxes keeps a woman from getting HIV during sex. T F DK
16. A woman can get HIV if she has anal sex with a man. T F DK
17. Showering or washing one's genitals after sex keeps a person from getting HIV. T F DK
18. A man can get HIV if he has vaginal sex with a woman who has HIV. T F DK
19. Eating healthy foods can keep a person from getting HIV. T F DK
20. All pregnant women infected with HIV will have babies born with AIDS. T F DK
21. Using a latex condom or rubber can lower a person's chance of getting HIV. T F DK
22. Taking a birth control pill keeps a woman from getting HIV. T F DK
23. A diaphragm and a birth control pill provide the same protection against HIV infection. T F DK
24. Most people with AIDS will die from it. T F DK
25. A person with HIV can look and feel healthy. T F DK

26. There are more cases of HIV in the USA than in the rest of the world. T F DK
27. People who have been infected with HIV quickly show serious signs of being infected. T F DK
28. A person can be infected with HIV for 5 years or more without getting AIDS. T F DK
29. There is a vaccine that can stop adults from getting AIDS. T F DK
30. Some drugs have been made for the treatment of AIDS. T F DK
31. There is a blood test to tell if a person has been infected with HIV. T F DK
32. Women are always tested for HIV during their pap smears. T F DK
33. A person cannot get HIV by having oral sex, mouth to penis, with a man who has HIV. T F DK
34. In the USA, most cases of AIDS have resulted from sex between men and women. T F DK
35. A person can get HIV even if she or he has sex with another person only one time. T F DK
36. A mother with HIV can pass it on to her baby by breast-feeding. T F DK
37. Using a lambskin condom or rubber is the best protection against HIV. T F DK
38. An undetectable viral load means that HIV is gone from the body. T F DK

39. People are likely to get HIV by deep kissing, putting their tongue in their partner's mouth, if their partner has HIV. T F DK
40. Infection with HIV leads to AIDS. T F DK
41. A person can get HIV by giving blood. T F DK
42. A woman cannot get HIV if she has sex during her period. T F DK
43. You can usually tell if someone has HIV by looking at them. T F DK
44. There is a female condom that can help decrease a woman's chances of getting HIV. T F DK
45. A natural skin condom works better against HIV than does a latex condom. T F DK
46. A person will NOT get HIV if she or he is taking antibiotics. T F DK
47. Having sex with more than one partner can increase a person's chance of being infected with HIV. T F DK
48. Taking a test for HIV one week after having sex will tell a person if she or he has HIV. T F DK
49. A person can get HIV by sitting in a hot tub or a swimming pool with a person who has HIV. T F DK
50. A person can get HIV through contact with saliva, tears, sweat, or urine. T F DK

51. A person can get HIV from a woman's vaginal secretions (wetness from her vagina). T F DK

52. A person is more likely to get HIV if she or he has another STD (VD), such as herpes or the clap. T F DK

53. Taking the AIDS drug, AZT, lowers the chance of a pregnant woman with HIV giving it to her baby. T F DK

54. Outside of the USA, most cases of AIDS have resulted because of IV (needle) drug use or men having sex with men. T F DK

55. A person can get HIV if having oral sex, mouth on vagina, with a woman. T F DK

56. If a person tests positive for HIV, then the test site will have to tell all of his or her partners. T F DK

57. Using Vaseline or baby oil with condoms lowers the chance of getting HIV. T F DK

58. Washing drug use equipment with cold water kills HIV. T F DK

59. A woman can get HIV if she has vaginal sex with a man who has HIV. T F DK

60. Athletes who share needles when using steroids can get HIV from the needles. T F DK

61. Douching after sex will keep a woman from getting HIV. T F DK

62. Taking vitamins keeps a person from getting HIV. T F DK

1

What Are HIV and AIDS?

Hundreds of people had fallen ill and many people had died before HIV was first identified. The virus that causes AIDS is an elusive enemy, differing from most other viruses in that it hides throughout the body. Fortunately, scientists have discovered much about HIV and how it causes AIDS.

The Virus That Causes AIDS

Because HIV is a virus, understanding its nature starts with a basic understanding of viruses in general. All viruses share important features in common. A *virus* consists of a small strand of genetic material (DNA or RNA) encased within a protective covering or coat. A virus is not a cell and does not have any of the essential parts of living cells. It can be described as something between an inanimate object and a living organism. A virus invades a cell and takes control of its functions; it uses the cell's own resources to recreate itself and to make millions of new virus particles. Unlike living cells, a virus does not have a life of its own; a virus is able to survive and reproduce only when it is inside a living cell. Although symptoms caused by viruses can often be treated, viral infections are difficult to cure. HIV is a member of a group of viruses called *retroviruses* that are unique in the way that they infect cells and cause disease.

How are viruses different from bacteria?

Infections that lead to illness in humans have many causes. Bacteria, for example, are a common cause of disease. *Bacteria* are tiny single-cell organisms that invade the body, disrupt the workings of cells, and cause sickness. A big difference between viral and bacterial infections is that bacterial infections can usually be treated and cured with antibiotics. Examples of bacterial infections include strep throat and salmonella food poisoning, and examples of sexually transmitted bacterial infections include gonorrhea and syphilis. All of these infections can be treated and cured with antibiotics.

Viruses are much smaller than bacteria. An example of a common sexually transmitted virus is herpes simplex virus, which infects nerve endings and mucous membranes. Thus, both bacteria and viruses attack body cells to cause disease, but they do so in very different ways.

What is HIV?

HIV is the virus that causes AIDS. The letters *HIV* stand for *human immunodeficiency virus*:

- Human, because it infects only human beings
- Immunodeficiency, because it attacks and destroys the body's immune system
- Virus, because it shares biological characteristics with other viruses that are not common to living cells.

What kind of virus is HIV?

HIV is a *retrovirus*. As the name suggests, the life cycle of a retrovirus is the reverse of other viruses, making it far more difficult to understand than common viruses. HIV belongs to a group of retroviruses called *lentiviruses* (*lenti* means "slow" in Latin) because it progresses slowly; it usually takes years before symptoms appear. HIV is an infection of the immune system, the very system that the body uses to fend off infections. The outer envelope of HIV consists of lipids, or fats, and glycoproteins, such as gp120 and gp44. The glycoproteins play a critical role in determining how HIV attaches itself to immune cells. Inside the envelope is HIV's genetic core, which consists of a strand of RNA. The core also has three important enzymes: reverse transcriptase, protease, and integrase. These enzymes are essential to the process by which HIV replicates itself and produces new virus inside of immune cells.

How does HIV infect blood?

The target of HIV is a specific type of white blood cells called *T-helper lymphocyte cells* or just *T-helper cells*. T-helper cells control several branches of the immune system. T-helper cells are like the generals of the body's army, commanding other immune cells to destroy possible causes of infection and disease. By killing T-helper cells, HIV disables the entire immune system. HIV attaches itself to the lymphocyte cell surface at an area called the *CD4 receptor site*, the location on the T-helper cell that HIV uses to gain entry to the T-helper cell. Infected T-helper cells are rendered defenseless against HIV. Over time, T-helper cells are destroyed by HIV, profoundly impairing the body's ability to fight off many diseases. Even before they are killed, infected T-helper cells, as well as other immune cells called *monocytes* and *macrophages*, lose their ability to fight infections and prevent disease. The immune system attempts to control HIV by producing antibodies against the virus. Unfortunately, these efforts are only partly effective, because HIV hides inside of T-helper cells, slowly infecting more and more cells until the entire immune system itself can no longer function.

Is there more than one virus that causes AIDS?

There are two known types of HIV. The first type is referred to as *HIV type-1*, or just *HIV-1*, which accounts for the majority of AIDS cases in the world and almost all AIDS cases in the United States. A second AIDS-causing virus, *HIV-2*, was discovered in 1986 and is common to some areas of East Africa. In terms of their biological makeup, HIV-1 and HIV-2 are more alike than they are different: Both are retroviruses and both cause AIDS. However, the two viruses are quite different in the rate at which they destroy the immune system: HIV-1 destroys T-helper cells more quickly than does HIV-2. In addition, HIV-2 has not spread geographically at nearly the rate of HIV-1. From here on, I use *HIV* to refer to HIV-1 unless otherwise noted.

What is the difference between HIV and AIDS?

HIV and AIDS have often been confused. HIV is the name of the virus that, when introduced into the human bloodstream, infects white blood cells that do much of the immune system's work to control disease. A person who is infected with HIV does not necessarily feel sick. In fact, people usually feel healthy for years after they have become infected with HIV. As HIV infection progresses, the immune system slowly breaks down, leaving the person vulnerable to other diseases that are normally fought off by a healthy immune system. AIDS is the later stage of HIV infection. A person is diagnosed with AIDS after the immune system becomes disabled by HIV or when the person becomes seriously ill from diseases that take advantage of the broken-down immune system.

What is the HIV cycle?

Every virus has a cycle, the course by which it multiplies and spreads. A virus cycle is like a life cycle, except that a virus does not have a life of its own. So a virus is dependent on living cells for its replication cycle. In most viral infections, a virus places its DNA genetic material into a cell to take over its resources and manufacture more viruses. For HIV, the cycle is reversed from the usual biological sequence, causing one of the most perplexing aspects of HIV infection. The first step in the HIV cycle occurs when the virus attaches itself to the CD4 receptor site on the outer surface of the immune cell. The virus injects its inner core of RNA—another form of genetic material—and an enzyme called *reverse transcriptase*, the enzyme that transforms viral RNA core into DNA. The transformed viral DNA enters the cell nucleus, where the cell DNA exists. The viral genetic material then weaves itself together with the cell DNA to form what is called a *pro-virus*. The new combined DNA now includes the virus material and directs the cell to assemble and release more HIV. The enzyme protease plays an important part in assembling new HIV particles. When it is released, the multiplied HIV goes on to infect more cells, repeating the HIV viral cycle.

How has HIV become such a devastating disease?

HIV has become the world's greatest threat to public health for many reasons. First, HIV is transmitted from person to person; individuals with HIV infect their sex partners and needle-sharing partners, often without knowing that they themselves are infected. Second, HIV infection eventually leads to AIDS and death. Third, there is no known cure for HIV infection. Fourth, international travel, now commonplace, has allowed HIV to rapidly spread across the world. Finally, HIV is spread through common sexual behaviors and addictive drug behaviors that are difficult for people to change.

What makes HIV so difficult to fight?

HIV infiltrates the command and control centers of the immune system, attacking the very cells that would normally fight it off. HIV incorporates itself into the cells, where it remains hidden for a long time, eventually replicating itself and destroying the host cells. Attempts to directly kill HIV can destroy the very immune cells that must be saved. Another problem with fighting HIV is that the virus rapidly changes itself, mutating while it continues to infect new cells. Mutations make it difficult to develop a vaccine against HIV. Also, mutations can be resistant to anti-HIV medications, making it more difficult to treat the virus.

How many different strains of HIV are there?

Genetic analyses have suggested that HIV-1 stems from a single virus that originated sometime between 1920 and 1950. Research that has examined the gene sequences of HIV has categorized HIV-1 into two major groups, designated by the letters M and O, and each group is further broken down into subtypes, with 10 subtypes of the M group. The different genetic subtypes of HIV are distributed differently across regions of the world, with the M subtypes accounting for nearly all HIV infections in North and South America. Subtle genetic variations, or mutations, within any given type or subtype of HIV result in great genetic diversity and therefore many different strains.

What does it mean that HIV mutates?

Mutations are genetic alterations and errors that occur when cells as well as viruses reproduce. Cell mutations are usually infrequent mistakes that do not cause serious problems. Mutations are also a regular part of the cycle of retroviruses, including HIV. As a retrovirus, HIV mutates rapidly, so it develops into many strains, each slightly different from the others. Some strains produce disease slowly and others more quickly; more rapidly destructive viruses are called *virulent strains*. Virulent strains of HIV create major obstacles to treating HIV infection and make it extremely difficult to create an effective vaccine. HIV also mutates in response to medications designed to suppress its replication activity, allowing the virus to develop resistance to anti-HIV drugs and ultimately rendering these treatments ineffective. Mutated HIV gives rise to a greater variety of the virus, but each mutation is nevertheless a part of the HIV family. Because the most basic characteristics of the virus do not mutate, HIV is not changing into a different virus that could spread in new and different ways.

How is HIV different from human T-cell lymphotropic virus (HTLV) type-I and HTLV-II?

HIV, HTLV-I, and HTLV-II are similar in that they are all human retroviruses containing RNA and reverse transcriptase. All three are carried in the blood and other body fluids, and all three infect white blood cells. Scientists who discovered the first human retrovirus, HTLV-I, originally named the virus that causes AIDS HTLV-III, the third human retrovirus. However, today HIV and the HTLVs are considered distinct viruses. HTLV-I can cause leukemia, cancer of white blood cells (leukocytes). HTLV-II seems related to leukemia, but its role in disease is not well understood. HIV, on the other hand, causes AIDS. Although HTLV and HIV both disable white blood cells, the resulting diseases are different. Leukemia results in rapid and uncontrolled growth of white blood cells, whereas HIV infection systematically kills white blood cells. Thus, although they share some things in common, the HTLVs do not cause AIDS, and HIV does not cause leukemia.

Is HIV different from the viruses that cause hepatitis?

Yes. Hepatitis viruses cause serious liver disease, but they do not attack the body's immune system. Some hepatitis viruses are transmitted from person to person through sexual contact and through dirty injection needles, and this is particularly true of hepatitis B virus. HIV and hepatitis B virus are both common among men who have sex with men and people who inject drugs. People who have both HIV and hepatitis B infections may suffer severe liver disease caused by hepatitis B virus, which can worsen as HIV takes its toll on the immune system. Both HIV and hepatitis viruses can and often do infect the same person. But HIV and hepatitis infections are very different diseases. See Exhibit 1.1 for the diseases associated with common viruses.

Is HIV similar to the virus that causes herpes?

No. Herpes simplex viruses are not retroviruses. Herpes simplex viruses infect nerve endings and cause painful blisters on the mucous membranes at the site of infection. And unlike HIV, herpes simplex viruses do not infect the immune system.

Herpes and HIV are often confused for the following reasons:

1. Both herpes simplex virus and HIV are sexually transmitted infections, so people can get both diseases the same way.
2. Like HIV, herpes simplex virus can remain hidden without causing symptoms for months or years.
3. Herpes infections cause open blisters when the infection is active, and these openings in the skin

EXHIBIT 1.1. Common Viruses and the Diseases They Cause

Common virus	*Associated disease*
Human Papilloma Virus (HPV)	A very common sexually transmitted disease that causes genital warts but is often without symptoms. Difficult to treat, often recurrent.
Human Immunodeficiency Virus	Causes severe immune system disease that leads to AIDS.
Herpes Simplex Virus–Type 2	Causes painful blisters and inflammation of the nerve endings at the site of mucous membrane infection.
Cytomegalovirus (CMV)	Sexually and nonsexually transmitted, causes flulike symptoms. Can be serious in people with AIDS.
Epstein-Barr Virus	Causes mononucleosis—fever, sore throat, swollen lymph nodes.
Hepatitis Virus C	The hepatitis viruses can cause serious liver disease. Hepatitis C is spread by contact with blood of an infected person.

can increase the ability of HIV to be transmitted during sex.

4. A person with HIV infection who also has herpes usually experiences more frequent outbreaks of blisters when HIV degrades the immune system.

5. There is no known cure for either of these viral infections.

Despite these similarities, herpes simplex virus causes an entirely different disease than does HIV, it does not disable the immune system, and it does not cause AIDS.

The Origins of AIDS

Information about where in the world a disease started does not help us prevent, treat, or deal with it. Still, curiosity does serve an important purpose. Fear of the unknown can be immobilizing, so understanding where a disease came from may help people understand its cause and thus gain a sense of control.

When was the first case of AIDS identified?

The first cases of AIDS were documented in the spring of 1981. The Centers for Disease Control and Prevention (CDC) reported on June 5, 1981, that 5 young, previously healthy men in Los Angeles were hospitalized with a rare disease, pneumocystis carinii pneumonia. One month later, on July 3, another 10 men with the same type of pneumonia and 26 men with Kaposi's sarcoma, a rare form of skin cancer, were also reported by the CDC. These men lived in New York City, San Francisco, and Los Angeles and were young and gay. These clusters of previously healthy men with rare diagnoses caused alarm among public health officials and the medical community. Soon afterward, many more cases of AIDS were reported, and the disease soon became recognized as a global health threat.

How was HIV discovered?

When AIDS first spread across Europe and North America, its cause was completely unknown. People feared that AIDS was passed from person to person through casual contact. The worst fears were that a person could get AIDS through the air, like catching a cold or the flu. However, because the first cases of AIDS occurred almost exclusively among men who had sex with men and people who injected drugs, it was thought to be a disease transmitted by sexual and blood contact. Because of the seriousness of AIDS and the rapid increase in AIDS cases, scientists vigorously searched for its cause. Between 1983 and 1984, just 2 years after the first cases of AIDS were described, the virus that causes AIDS was discovered almost simultaneously by three independent laboratories and given three different names: *lymphadenopathy associated virus*, discovered by Luc Montagnier of the Pasteur Institute of France; *HTLV-III*, discovered by Robert Gallo at the National Cancer Institute in Washington, DC; and *AIDS-associated retrovirus*, discovered by Jay Levy of the Cancer Research Institute of the University of California at San Francisco.

It turned out that all three viruses were very similar and were actually variations of the same virus, which in 1986 was given the name *human immunodeficiency virus*.

Where did AIDS originally come from?

The earliest documented case of HIV infection occurred in 1959. The virus was isolated in a stored blood sample collected from a man in Kinshasa, Democratic Republic of Congo. How this man became infected is not known. The exact origin of AIDS is therefore not known, but there are several theories of how HIV came to be.

The theory of recent emergence states that AIDS has been around for hundreds of years but was isolated to remote areas of Africa and has only recently been recognized. However, this explanation is not well accepted because there is little evidence that anyone in the world was infected with HIV before 1950.

Mutation theory holds that HIV recently evolved through the mutation of another human virus. Scientists have dismissed this explanation because characteristics of HIV do not match up well with other human viruses, making it unlikely that HIV has a human virus ancestry.

Theories of biological accidents have been discussed, in which HIV is thought to have been introduced to people through a medical or biological mistake. One such theory is that HIV emerged from a contaminated batch of an oral polio vaccine administered in Central Africa in the middle part of the last century. These theories are very controversial.

The intestinal fluke "theory" suggests that HIV resides in a parasite of the thymus gland. When the parasite, or fluke, is removed, HIV and AIDS are cured. This theory has no scientific basis and promotes a false hope for an unproven cure.

Conspiracy theories state that HIV was developed as a biological weapon or as a means to eliminate entire segments of society. However, no evidence supports any such conspiracy or genocide theories.

The zoonosis theory is widely discussed as a possible origin of HIV. Zoonosis states that HIV stems from a related virus that infects certain African primates and that the virus only recently infected humans. The process of a virus moving from an animal species to humans is called *zoonosis* and is known to have occurred with other viruses. This explanation seems plausible because HIV is genetically similar to viruses that infect primates living in areas of Africa where HIV-1 is common. Still, zoonosis has not been entirely accepted as the origin of HIV.

It is most commonly agreed that HIV is a virus that developed in humans in Central Africa between the 1920s and 1950s and only recently spread because of migration and transcontinental travel. Exactly how HIV first emerged in humans is not known.

HIV in the Body

Infected T-helper cells and other infected cells of the immune system can contain millions of virus particles.

Transmission of HIV from one person to another therefore involves moving the virus from the bloodstream and other body fluids of one person to those of another. Infected blood, semen, or vaginal fluids must enter the body for HIV infection to occur.

Are people with certain blood types more susceptible to HIV infection than others?

No. Regardless of whether a person's blood type is A, B, AB, or O, and no matter if the blood type is RH+ or RH–, human blood can become infected with HIV. All human blood types contain immune cells that have the CD4 receptor site on their surface and are vulnerable to HIV infection. There is nothing special about a particular blood type that can protect it against HIV, nor is there anything that leads one blood type to more easily get infected.

If HIV is a blood disease, then why is it in vaginal fluids and semen?

HIV is found in large quantities in certain body fluids that are derived from blood. HIV infects immune system cells, particularly T-helper cells, monocytes, and macrophages, and these cells are found throughout the body. Moreover, immune cells that become infected with HIV are found in many body fluids derived from blood, particularly semen, pre-ejaculation fluids, breast milk, and vaginal secretions (see Exhibit 1.2).

EXHIBIT 1.2. HIV in Human Body Fluids

Body fluids with high concentrations of HIV	
Blood	Semen
Vaginal fluids	Breast milk
Body fluids with low or no concentrations of HIV	
Saliva	Sweat
Tears	Urine
Feces	

Is HIV in breast milk?

Yes, HIV is found in breast milk of women infected with the virus. T-helper, monocyte, and macrophage cells are common in breast milk because they provide immune protection. Babies born uninfected with HIV can become infected through breast-feeding from an infected woman.

Is HIV found in saliva?

Unless there is blood present, the amount of HIV in saliva is very small. Like other body fluids, saliva can contain HIV as well as HIV-infected immune system cells. However, HIV is not detectable in the saliva of many HIV-positive people.

Does saliva inactivate the virus?

Saliva contains chemicals that create a harsh environment for HIV and can inactivate the virus. However,

HIV often remains protected, hiding inside of its host immune cells. HIV is more prominent in saliva if blood is present, particularly when there is an open cut in the mouth or a person has an oral infection or gum disease.

What are the risks of getting HIV from saliva?

The likelihood of HIV infection from saliva has been controversial, to say the least. Because HIV is found in the saliva of some infected people, studies suggest that HIV can be transmitted through saliva when it comes in close contact with another person's bloodstream. However, most researchers have concluded that contact with the saliva of an HIV-infected person through kissing, CPR, or other means carries no risk for HIV infection.

The low risk of contact with saliva likely results because there are two conditions necessary for HIV transmission. First, there must be sufficient amounts of HIV present to allow infection. Although it is not known exactly what minimum dose of HIV is required for infection, saliva just doesn't seem to have enough virus present to cause infection. Second, there must be a point of exposure for HIV to infect cells that are susceptible to infection—access to immune cells that have CD4 receptor sites on their surfaces. Blood transfusions therefore cause infection in more than 90% of people who receive HIV-infected blood—immune cells in the blood are exposed to large amounts of HIV. In contrast, HIV infection from kissing is considered most improbable—few immune cells in the mouth are exposed to very little HIV.

Is HIV present in sweat, tears, urine, or feces?

The amount of HIV found in tears, urine, and feces is far less than amounts found in blood, semen, and vaginal fluids. HIV is not usually found in sweat. Contact with urine, feces, and tears is not known to constitute a risk for transmitting HIV infection because of the small amount of HIV present. However, other viruses, such as hepatitis B virus, can easily be spread through contact with saliva, urine, and feces.

Does contact with HIV-infected body fluids always result in infection?

No. HIV transmission does not occur as easily as it may seem. In theory, contact with HIV could result in HIV infection. In fact, however, HIV infection resulting from contact with any fluid other than infected blood, semen, vaginal fluids, or breast milk is virtually nonexistent. It is easy to forget that HIV is most concentrated in blood, semen, vaginal fluids, and breast milk and to focus on the more remote ways that a person could get infected. However, the reality is that there are only a few ways that people become infected with HIV, all of which involve sharing blood, semen, vaginal fluids, or breast milk. Even then, many factors can increase or decrease the risk for infection, many of which are not well understood.

HIV Outside the Body

Some viruses can be transmitted from person to person through coughing or sneezing without direct contact with body fluids. Whether a virus is able to infect someone through the air depends entirely on how durable the virus is outside of the body. Exposure to HIV through the air is a frightening thought because it implies that anyone can be infected at any time. Fortunately, HIV is not an airborne virus.

How long does HIV remain active outside the body?

HIV cannot remain active outside of the human body for very long. HIV is packaged in a delicate outer wrapping called an *envelope*. Some viruses have a tough outer protective *capsule*, but viruses like HIV that have an envelope are the least durable. Under the controlled conditions of a laboratory, HIV remains active in purified nonchlorinated water for several days. Unfortunately, these research findings can easily be misinterpreted. A common misconception is that HIV transmission can occur when drinking from the same glass used by a person who has AIDS or when swimming in a public pool. In fact, HIV is quickly destroyed in tap water and pool water. HIV's envelope is extremely sensitive to even mild chemicals, like detergents or small amounts of chlorine.

In a controlled laboratory, HIV can also survive on dry surfaces at room temperature. Again, in natural environments it is inconceivable that immune cells could be exposed to a sufficient amount of HIV through contact with the virus on surfaces like tabletops, toilet seats, or furniture. There is absolutely no evidence to suggest that a person can get HIV from touching inanimate objects or surfaces, or from touching people infected with HIV.

Can HIV be transmitted by contact with dried blood?

Dried blood from a person who is HIV positive can contain large amounts of active HIV. For example, dried blood contaminates injection needles and can cause infection when needles are shared. Direct contact with blood, dried or fresh, should always be avoided because of the potential for spread of many diseases including HIV. When cleaning dried blood, you should use detergent or bleach and wear plastic or rubber gloves.

Can HIV exist in the air?

No. HIV does not survive long when exposed directly to air. The environment inside the cells and body fluids protects the virus. However, when HIV is out of the safety of cells or body fluids, it is vulnerable and is rapidly degraded.

Do hot temperatures destroy HIV?

HIV is very sensitive to heat. Temperatures above 133°F (56°C) are considered hot enough to inactivate the virus. These temperatures are used to decontaminate biological products and pasteurize blood used in medical treatments. Boiling inactivates the virus even more quickly, allowing for proper sterilization of medical instruments to protect against contamination with HIV.

The AIDS Epidemic

Tracking the HIV/AIDS epidemic falls within the purview of local health departments, the CDC, and the World Health Organization (WHO). Public health surveillance closely monitors the number of people diagnosed with illnesses classified as AIDS. However, because it can take years for a person with HIV infection to develop AIDS, even the most accurate estimates of AIDS cases only approximate the seriousness of the HIV epidemic. Because only counting AIDS cases is so limited, it has become increasingly common for HIV infections to be reported and tracked, allowing for a more precise estimate of HIV infections.

How many people in the world are infected with HIV?

It is impossible to know the exact number of HIV infections. The WHO estimates that 34 million people in the world are living with HIV/AIDS. It is also estimated that 15 million adults and almost 4 million children in the world have died of AIDS. The most heavily AIDS-affected areas of the world are sub-Saharan Africa, South and Southeast Asia, Latin America, the Caribbean Islands, and North America, and these regions continue to have the highest rate of HIV infections. However, Africa carries the greatest burden of AIDS; 70% of people with HIV in the world live in sub-Saharan Africa. The WHO estimates that as many as 16,000 individuals are infected with HIV each day, and 90% of these new incidents occur in developing countries (see Figure 1.1 for the estimated number of HIV infections across regions of the world).

How many people in the United States are infected with HIV?

According to the best available information, nearly 1 million adults in the United States are infected with HIV, with as many as 40,000 to 80,000 new HIV infections occurring each year. Each year the number of AIDS cases in the United States increases. Figure 1.2 shows the rapid increase of AIDS cases in the United States. Each dot in the figures represents 30 cases of AIDS. In 1985 (Panel A) there was only a scattering of AIDS cases, with rapid growth in AIDS occurring during the late 1980s (Panel B) and an explosion across the United States during the 1990s (Panel C). It took more than 8 years

North America
900,000
Latin America
1.3 Million
Western Europe
520,000
Eastern Europe &
Central Asia
420,000
East Asia & Pacific
530,000
North Africa &
Middle East
220,000
South & Southeast Asia
5.6 Million
sub-Saharan Africa
24.5 Million
Australia &
New Zealand
15,000

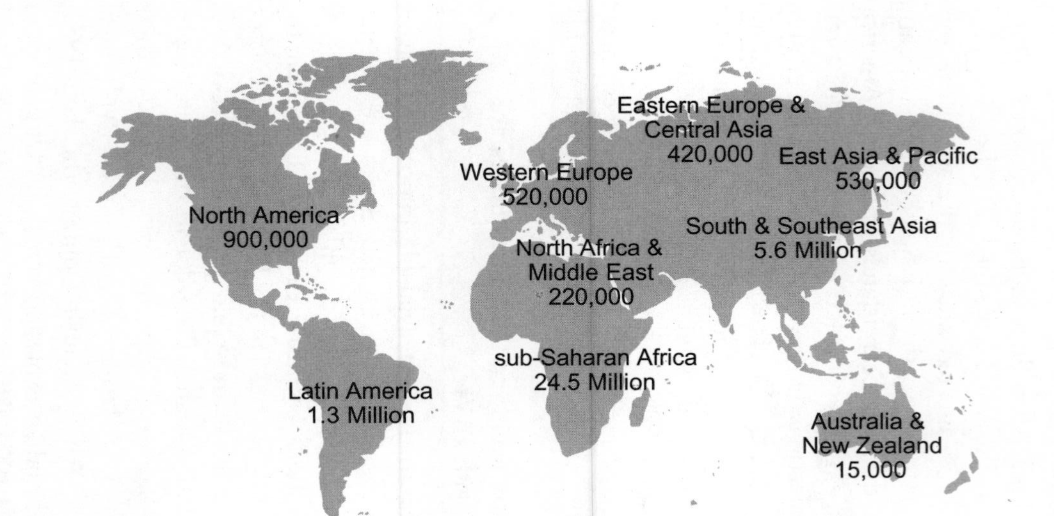

FIGURE 1.1. A global perspective on AIDS, 2001 (Source: UNAIDS, 2001).

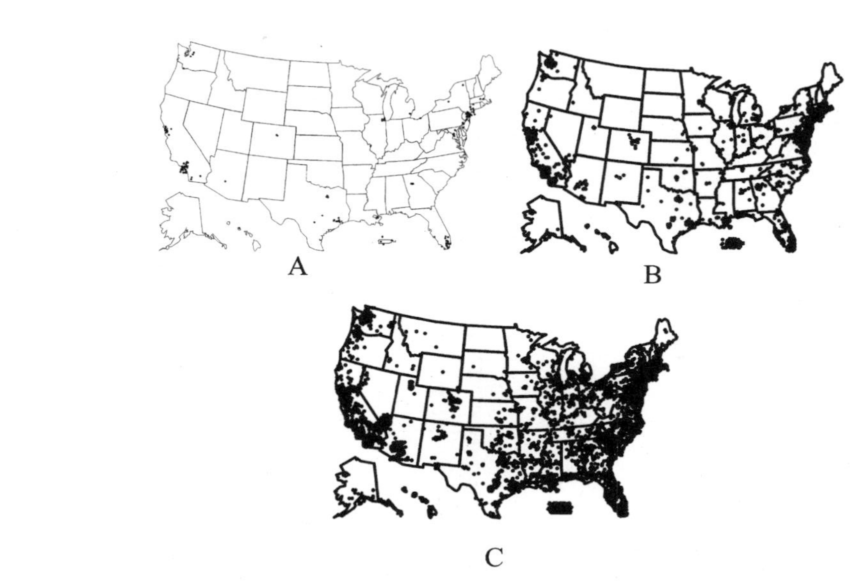

FIGURE 1.2. Cumulative AIDS cases in the United States in 1985 (A: 10,000 cases), 1989 (B: 100,000 cases), and 1995 (C: 500,000 cases). Each dot represents 30 cases of AIDS (Source: CDC, 2001).

for the first 100,000 cases of AIDS to occur in the United States, but the second 100,000 AIDS cases were reported in just 2 years. The third 100,000 cases occurred in less than 2 years, and the rapid increase of AIDS cases continued from that point forward. Figure 1.3 shows the rates of AIDS cases per 100,000 persons for each state in the United States as of midyear 2000.

How many people have died from AIDS in the United States?

As of 1999, 196,000 men, 41,000 women, and 2,500 children had died of AIDS in the United States, making AIDS the leading cause of death among young men and women in several large cities and accounting for 1 in 3 deaths among young adults in some U.S. cities. However, because of advances in the treatment of HIV and AIDS, the number of people dying of AIDS-related causes has declined in recent years even though greater numbers of people continue to be diagnosed with AIDS.

Are people with AIDS living longer today than in the past?

Yes. Many people who have access to anti-HIV medications are living longer than ever before. New cases of AIDS have increased each year, whereas the number of AIDS deaths has decreased, making the prevalence of people living with AIDS greater each year. Given

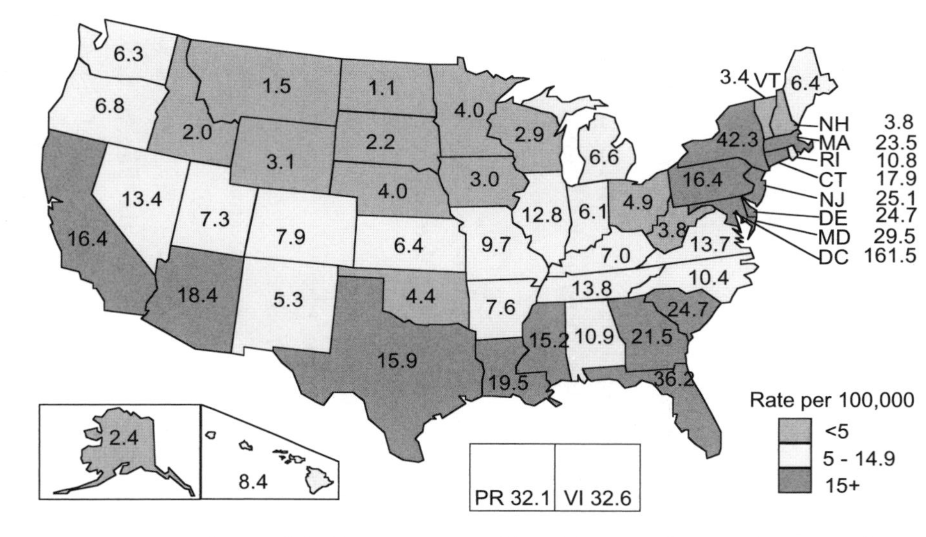

FIGURE 1.3. Rates of AIDS cases reported in U.S. states (Source: CDC, 2001).

the growing number of people with AIDS in the United States and the continued advances in HIV treatment, people with AIDS are expected to continue to live longer than was possible in the past. However, the majority of people living with AIDS in the world do not have access to anti-HIV medications, and they face the ravages of untreated HIV.

Are people in certain places in the United States more affected by AIDS than others?

Throughout the epidemic, AIDS in the United States has mostly occurred in major cities on the East and West Coasts, and this has been true throughout the epidemic. With most people infected with HIV living in larger cities, AIDS resembles other epidemics in the history of the world, including the Black Plague, which ravaged 14th-century Europe. In the United States, HIV first occurred among men who have sex with men and people who inject drugs, particularly those living in New York City, Los Angeles, and San Francisco, and it spread outward from the cities. Thus, states with the greatest incidence of AIDS span the coast of California, along the U.S.–Mexican border, along the Gulf states, and up the Eastern Seaboard. States along the U.S.–Canadian border and in the nation's midsection have the least number of AIDS cases. Today, AIDS is growing in rural areas and threatens to become a rural as well as an urban health crisis.

Have men and women been equally affected by AIDS?

In North America, more men have been diagnosed with AIDS than women, primarily because gay and bisexual men have been affected the most and for the longest time. However, it is a much different story in other parts of the world. In Africa, for example, HIV is primarily heterosexually transmitted with greater risks to women than to men because HIV is more easily transmitted in the female reproductive tract and HIV-positive men are more likely to have multiple female partners.

What ethnic groups have been most affected by AIDS?

In the United States, half of all AIDS cases have occurred among White people, one third among African Americans, and most of the rest of the cases among Hispanics, with a smaller number among Asian Americans, Pacific Islanders, and Native Americans. At first it appears that White people have been the most seriously affected by AIDS, but the absolute numbers of people living with AIDS are deceptive. Considering that African Americans make up less than 15% and Hispanics less than 15% of the total U.S. population, HIV has obviously disproportionally affected racial and ethnic minorities (see Figure 1.4). Another indicator of the impact of HIV on minorities is that most HIV-infected newborns in New York City are born to

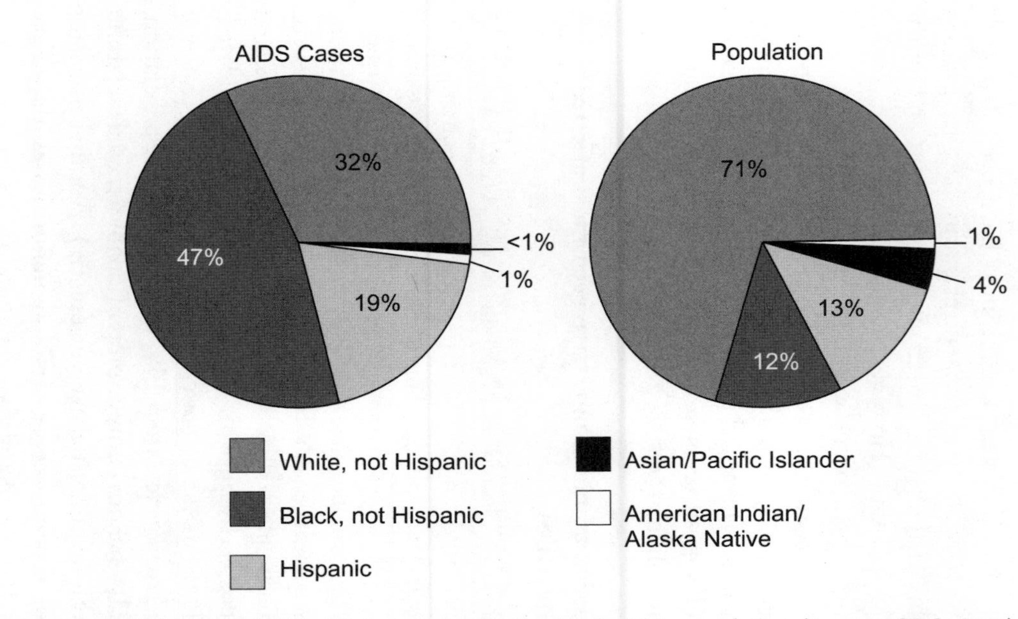

FIGURE 1.4. Ethnicity of U.S. AIDS cases in relation to the U.S. population (Source: CDC, 2001).

minority women. Because HIV is transmitted from person to person through intimate contact, the more people with HIV infection who have unprotected sexual intercourse in a given place at a given time, the greater the likelihood of the virus spreading.

Who is most likely to get AIDS?

Only people with HIV infection will get AIDS. What people do, not who they are, determines whether they get the virus. HIV infection results from behaviors that expose an uninfected person's bloodstream or mucus membranes to the blood, semen, or vaginal fluids of an infected person. People who engage in fluid-exchanging sexual behavior or who share needles to inject drugs with an HIV-infected partner account for the vast majority of people who become HIV infected and eventually get AIDS.

Summary

HIV was discovered in 1983, and it quickly became apparent that HIV infects people and causes disease in complex ways. Ultimately, HIV causes AIDS, and the disease progresses fastest when it is left untreated. Having HIV infection does not necessarily mean that a person feels sick. It takes years for the virus to disable the immune system. It is only after the destruction of the immune system that a person with HIV becomes ill. Questions about HIV infection and how it causes AIDS are answered in chapter 2.

2

How Does HIV Cause AIDS?

Infections cause disease by disrupting normal body processes. HIV causes a particularly devastating disease because it infects the very cells that normally fight off viruses. Destruction of the body's immune system leaves a person vulnerable to many life-threatening diseases. The disabling of the body's defenses against disease is the essence of AIDS. This chapter answers questions about HIV disease and how it causes AIDS.

The First Stages

A virus is dependent on living cells for its own survival. Some viruses are able to live in harmony with their host cell, using their host for their own needs without killing the cell or causing disease. However, HIV genetically reprograms the cells to become virus-producing factories, a process that ultimately leads to the demise of the infected cells. HIV most profoundly affects cells that manage the human immune system, which makes HIV-positive people susceptible to a vari-

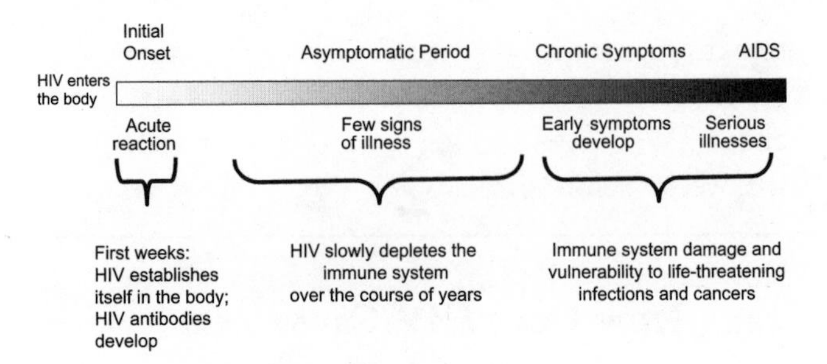

FIGURE 2.1. Stages of HIV infection.

ety of diseases against which they normally would have a defense. HIV infection therefore begins with the virus establishing itself inside the immune cells (and other cells that derive from immune cells, including certain cells in the nervous system and mucous membranes) and then progressing along a slow and relentless path of destruction until the person eventually succumbs to life-threatening illnesses. Figure 2.1 shows the stages of HIV infection from initial onset of the infection through the development of AIDS and can be useful in answering the questions that follow.

How long does it take for the body to show symptoms after initial exposure to HIV?

Soon after HIV enters the bloodstream, the immune system produces antibodies to fight the infection. Within a few months, these antibodies build up to a level that can be detected by an HIV antibody test. A person infected with HIV may also experience symptoms as part of the body's initial fight against infection. Acute early symptoms of HIV infection usually take about 2 to 4 weeks to appear and usually only last a few weeks before subsiding.

How can you tell if a person has been infected with HIV?

You cannot tell whether a person has HIV by looking at that person. People with HIV infection look and feel healthy for years after becoming infected. When the first symptoms of HIV do appear, they can resemble the flu. However, not everyone infected with HIV experiences these early symptoms. It usually takes a medical doctor who is familiar with treating HIV and AIDS to recognize the earliest symptoms of HIV when they do occur. The only way that even doctors can be sure whether a person has HIV is by administering an HIV antibody test.

If a person had a sexual encounter a year ago in which he or she may have contracted HIV, what are the chances that that person has not yet produced HIV antibodies?

Antibodies are part of the body's defensive response to HIV and are produced after HIV is detected by the immune system. The process that builds up antibodies in the bloodstream is called *seroconversion*—converting from HIV negative to HIV positive. Seroconversion can occur within 2 weeks of infection but can also take as long as several months. However, it is rare for a person to be infected with HIV for more than 6 months without producing HIV antibodies. The average person develops detectable HIV antibodies slightly more than 2 months after becoming infected, and almost everyone infected with HIV develops antibodies within 6 months. However, in very rare cases it can take longer than 6 months to develop detectable levels of HIV antibodies. The period between HIV infection and seroconversion is called the *window period;* a person can test HIV negative but still have the virus and be able to pass it to others during this time.

How long does it take for a person to get AIDS after testing positive for HIV antibodies?

The time it takes for a person to get AIDS after testing HIV positive depends mostly on the length of time between infection and testing and whether the person is receiving HIV treatments. AIDS is the end stage of HIV infection. It usually takes about 10 years—give or take 5 years—for a person with HIV to get AIDS. Effective HIV treatments can delay the onset of AIDS for several years. However, many people are hesitant to get tested, either because they do not think that they are infected or because they know they are at risk but are afraid to know the results. It is unfortunate that many people who do test positive for HIV antibodies do not get tested until they already have symptoms. Some people who test HIV positive already have an

AIDS-related illness when they first get tested. Getting tested later rather than sooner can reduce the potential long-term benefits of HIV treatments.

Can't the virus stay dormant in the body for years and not be detected?

It is true that HIV can remain dormant inside cells. At any given time, however, some of the HIV particles may be dormant while others are actively multiplying. To some degree, HIV is always replicating, even when a person has no symptoms. Detection of the virus depends on the body's antibody response to HIV, not activity of the virus itself. Even though HIV can remain hidden inside of cells, the immune system still produces antibodies against the virus, which can then be detected by an HIV antibody test.

Do some ways of getting HIV cause people to get AIDS sooner?

Early research suggested that people infected with HIV by certain modes of transmission lived longer than those infected through other modes of transmission. However, we now know that there are many possible explanations for these early research findings. For example, it is possible that people who inject drugs have additional health problems related to their drug abuse that may cause them to get ill sooner. People who get HIV from blood transfusions, including people with hemophilia and other blood diseases, have health problems that are not directly related to HIV that could cause a faster course of illness. Specific modes of HIV transmission no longer seem important in determining when a person with HIV develops AIDS.

Can someone with HIV get sick or die before the person who gave it to them?

Yes. Everyone's immune system is different and reacts differently to HIV. How healthy a person is when he or she becomes infected can influence the progression of HIV disease. Several other factors or cofactors can cause HIV infection to progress at a faster pace, such as the existence of other infections including some sexually transmitted infections and infection with specific strains or multiple strains of HIV. It is therefore possible for a person to develop AIDS before the person who transmitted the infection does, and in fact this often happens.

Do other viruses and diseases cause HIV infection to progress faster?

Yes, other infections can speed up the course of HIV disease. The effects of other viruses on HIV are considered particularly important because they may stimulate HIV that lies dormant inside the immune cells. One reason is that HIV becomes activated and starts reproducing itself when T-helper lymphocyte cells respond to other infections. Infections with combinations of viruses can also join forces or synergize to further increase the progression of HIV infection. Viruses that appear most important in stimulating HIV include hepatitis B; cytomegalovirus (CMV); and the family of herpes viruses, including herpes simplex and herpes zoster.

Can a person be a carrier for HIV?

No. In common terms, a *carrier* is a person who has the cause of a disease but does not develop the disease itself. Several viruses can be carried without causing illness, including herpes simplex viruses, CMV, and HTLV-I. Because it takes years before a person with HIV eventually becomes ill, people in the early stages of HIV infection could mistakenly be thought of as carriers, testing positive for HIV antibodies and without experiencing symptoms. Less than 10% of people with HIV infection remain symptom free for more than 10 years. Because everyone with HIV eventually appears to succumb to the active progression of the virus, people who have asymptomatic HIV infection cannot be regarded as carriers.

What is the incubation period for HIV?

An *incubation period* is the silent phase of an infection, the time between infection and the onset of disease processes and symptoms. For HIV, incubation occurs between infection and the onset of AIDS, which may be as long as 10 years in untreated people. For people receiving treatment, the HIV disease process is slowed, which extends the incubation period. During HIV incubation, large amounts of the virus are manufactured, and the immune system responds by producing antibodies.

What are the earliest symptoms that a person gets after they are infected with HIV?

The first symptoms of HIV infection are generally referred to as *acute HIV symptom illness* or *primary HIV infection*. Acute symptoms can include persistent fever, fatigue, muscle weakness, headache, meningitis (inflammation of membranes surrounding the brain), pain in or around the eyes, sensitivity to bright lights, sore throat, and skin rashes. Swollen lymph nodes (lymphadenopathy) are also common in the first few weeks of HIV infection. When acute symptoms do occur they usually last a short time, often less than a couple of weeks. See Exhibit 2.1 for the early symptoms of HIV infection.

Is the flu related to the early stages of HIV infection?

The acute symptoms of HIV infection, including fever, fatigue, muscle weakness, headache, and sore throat, can resemble the flu. However, there is no actual connection between the flu and HIV infection. Also, there is no evidence that people at the early stages of HIV infection get the flu more often than noninfected indi-

EXHIBIT 2.1. Early Symptoms of HIV Infection

- Sudden loss of weight
- Dry cough
- Recurring fever
- Night sweats
- Swollen lymph nodes in neck, armpits, or groin
- Diarrhea lasting more than 1 week
- White spots on tongue, mouth, or throat
- Pneumonia

viduals or that the flu is more serious in people with early HIV infection.

Are acute HIV symptoms the same as mononucleosis?

No, but acute symptoms of HIV infection are similar to the vague symptoms of mononucleosis. In particular, acute HIV symptoms can include swollen glands, which are often a part of mononucleosis. Primary HIV infection is an illness and is distinct from other infections.

If a person tests negative for HIV but gets sick, is it possible that he or she has HIV that has gone undetected?

It is possible for a person to test negative for HIV and still develop acute symptoms of HIV infection. The earliest symptoms of HIV infection usually occur, if at all, when antibodies against the virus are produced. Remember that a person who is tested after being exposed to HIV but before the body produces HIV antibodies still tests HIV negative. Therefore, it is possible for a person to get infected with HIV, test negative for HIV antibodies shortly after being infected, and then have acute symptoms.

The Silent Stages: HIV Infected and Feeling Fine

After the early symptoms of an acute HIV response subside, HIV continues to slowly destroy the immune system without any symptoms. This stage of HIV infection is called *asymptomatic HIV infection*; it is the time when a person has HIV infection and is symptom free.

What is the HIV latency period?

HIV latency refers to the period of time during which the virus remains inside the cells without reproducing itself. Latent infection occurs while HIV's genetic material (RNA) is integrated with the cell's own genetic material (DNA). Viral latency should not, however, be confused with the asymptomatic infection period. HIV is often actively reproducing itself during asymptomatic periods, and HIV can also be latent when a person is experiencing symptoms.

Can a person have HIV and look and feel healthy?

Yes. People with HIV infection generally look, feel, and are otherwise healthy. This is because the virus takes years to erode the immune system to a point at which they become vulnerable to disease.

Can HIV remain in the body for years without symptoms?

Yes, a person can be completely symptom free for years after being infected with HIV. However, even when a person is not showing symptoms, the virus remains in T-helper cells of the immune system where it actively depletes the immune system. During the long period without symptoms, the virus is disseminated throughout the body. In this state, it is also transmittable to others who are exposed to infected blood, semen, or vaginal fluids.

What is a T-helper cell count?

T-helper cells are one of several types of white blood cells that form the core of the immune system. *T* stands for thymus, the gland in the upper thorax or neck where T-helper cells mature after originating in bone marrow. There are three types of T-cells:

- *T-suppressor cells* provide feedback on the activity of the immune system and keep immune responses in check to prevent excessive immunity.

- *Cytotoxic T-cells* attack and destroy infected and cancer cells.
- *T-helper cells* link the branches of the immune system and manage immunity.

T-helper cells are the only ones among the three types to have CD4 receptor sites on their surface, making them susceptible to HIV infection. Reduction in the number of T-helper cells is an important way of tracking the progress of HIV infection. (T-helper count, T-cell count, and CD4 count are all names for the same test.) A count of the number of T-helper cells is often used to monitor the progression of HIV: Fewer T-helper cells mean more advanced HIV infection.

A common method of examining immune system decline is to count the number of T-helper lymphocyte cells in a specific unit of blood (a cubic millimeter). It is also common for doctors to examine the number of T-helper cells in relation to T-suppressor cells. T-suppressor cells regulate the immune system by not allowing immune cells to destroy healthy self-cells when protecting against disease. T-helper and T-suppressor cells therefore usually keep the immune system in balance. For healthy people who do not have an immune system disease, the number of T-helper cells is usually double the number of T-suppressor cells. However, with advanced HIV infection, the number of T-suppressor cells becomes greater than the declining number of T-helper cells. Eventually T-suppressor cells outnumber T-helper cells, signaling a failing immune system.

What is a normal T-helper cell count?

A normal T-helper cell count can vary greatly from person to person. Healthy adults usually have T-helper cell counts between 600 and 1,200 cells per unit of blood, with the average being about 1,000. Monitoring T-helper cell counts over a long time allows doctors to watch for patterns of increasing and decreasing numbers of cells. For people who have HIV, a drop in the number of T-helper cells means that HIV infection may be progressing.

What does it mean to have a low T-helper cell count?

A low T-helper cell count means different things for different people, depending on each individual's unique immune system. People become vulnerable to infections and other diseases when their T-helper cells drop below 200. When an HIV-positive person has a T-helper cell count of less than 200 cells per unit of blood, that person is diagnosed with AIDS.

How are T-helper cell counts related to the stages of HIV infection?

Most systems for diagnosing people at different points of HIV infection have an early stage, during which T-helper cell counts are typically greater than 500; a middle stage, during which people become vulnerable to some illnesses and T-helper cell counts fall between

500 and 200 cells per unit of blood; AIDS, when T-helper counts are less than 200; and later stages of AIDS, when T-helper cell counts are less than 100 and when people usually experience serious illnesses. However, because T-helper cell counts can fluctuate within a certain range, T-helper cell counts must be considered only one indicator of HIV disease progression.

Can a person have a low T-helper cell count and not be sick?

Yes. As T-helper cells decline, a person does become increasingly vulnerable to disease. Most infections and cancers related to AIDS occur when T-helper cells fall below 200 cells per unit of blood, and people with T-helper counts under 50 are often in poor health. Even people with less than 10 and even some people without any T-helper cells can go without illness for a long time. People are living longer and in better health with fewer T-helper cells because medications are now available to help prevent illnesses associated with AIDS.

What causes fluctuations in T-helper cell counts?

The number of T-helper cells circulating in blood can fluctuate greatly for any given individual. Even during the course of a day, the number of T-helper cells per unit of blood may fluctuate dramatically. The number of T-helper cells in the bloodstream also varies from morning to night and depends on whether the person has any type of infection. The lack of stability of T-helper cell counts can be a source of anxiety and worry for people with HIV infection because a drop in T-helper cells can signal that HIV infection is advancing. To minimize the amount of variation in T-helper cell counts, a person with HIV should

- wait about 3 weeks after recovering from an illness before having blood drawn,
- have blood drawn regularly at the same time of day, and
- use the same laboratory each time.

No single T-helper cell count should be taken as a clear sign that a person is getting better or worse. Rather, it is the pattern of T-helper cell counts over time that is most informative for projecting a person's changing health.

What is a viral load?

Viral load is an important tool for monitoring the activity of HIV in a person's body. *Viral load tests* measure the amount of HIV genetic material (RNA) present in blood or other body fluids. Viral load tests answer the question "how much HIV is present in a sample of blood?" This is an important question because the amount of HIV present is an important indicator of HIV disease progression. The greater the amount of HIV RNA present, or the greater the viral burden, the more active the virus is in replicating and therefore the more rapidly advancing the disease is in destroying the immune system. Today, viral load is used as a way to monitor the effectiveness of HIV treatments.

What does it mean to have an undetectable viral load?

Viral load tests have become increasingly more sensitive over the years since they first became available in 1996, with tests now able to detect very small quantities of HIV genetic material. However, every viral load test has its limits. A viral load test result that does not indicate any HIV RNA is said to be "undetectable" because the quantity of HIV RNA is so low that the test does not register. However, this does not mean that HIV is no longer present or that the person is no longer able to transmit the virus to others. An undetectable viral load test result is a positive sign in terms of one's health, but it does not mean that a person is cured.

When is a person's viral load at its highest?

HIV replicates itself rapidly at the earliest stages of HIV infection and at the later stages when a person has AIDS. However, viral load can be high during the course of HIV infection as well, especially when a person is not receiving anti-HIV medications.

What does a log viral load mean?

Viral load test results indicate how much virus is present as a result of the multiplication of the virus. Doctors use a transformation of the actual quantity of virus detected—or copies per milliliter (ml) of blood—which can range from less than 50 to a million. When values of viral load are large, it is difficult to interpret changes in absolute numbers of copies of viral load. It is therefore common to transform the viral load value to a log value. By transforming viral loads using a logarithmic (base 10) mathematical transformation, differences between values are more meaningful in terms of amount of HIV present. For example, if a log value is 5.0, then the number of HIV copies per ml in blood is 5.0 $\log_{10} = 10^5$copies/ml = 100,000 copies/ml.

What are the different tests of HIV viral load?

Several different laboratory techniques are available for testing HIV viral load. The most common technique is polymerase chain reaction (PCR); other techniques include branched-DNA signal amplification (b-DNA) and nucleic acid sequence-based amplification (NASBA). Each of these techniques is effective at detecting HIV genetic material, and each is commonly used depending on specific circumstances and laboratories. However, these tests all measure the amount of HIV genetic material in blood to gauge the progression of HIV disease and the effects of HIV treatments.

How long does it take for a person to get AIDS?

There just isn't a definite answer to this question. A minority of patients seem to move on a fast track from HIV infection to AIDS; they experience significant loss of T-helper cells within 1 to 2 years after getting infected and are diagnosed with AIDS shortly thereafter. In contrast, there are people who do not develop AIDS even after more than a decade of being diagnosed as HIV positive. These two extremes, however, are exceptions. As medical treatments for HIV advance, people tend to live longer with HIV infection and progress more slowly to AIDS. It is best to think of AIDS itself as a process rather than an event. It is not so much a matter of when a person gets AIDS but rather how the entire disease unfolds uniquely for each individual.

Symptoms of HIV Infection

Health is usually measured by the absence or presence of illness. The onset of the first symptoms of HIV ushers in the first sense of illness even after a person has been infected with HIV for a long time. There can be a sudden recognition that the virus is taking its toll on the body's ability to fight disease. For people who become ill but have not yet been tested, symptoms of HIV often sound an alarm that finally prompts them to get tested.

How long does it take for HIV symptoms to appear?

Following long periods of HIV infection, illness symptoms eventually develop. The earliest symptoms of HIV infection are often vague and include fever, swollen glands, and fatigue. T-helper cell counts usually drop below 500 T-helper cells per unit of blood when symptoms appear, but they rebound to normal levels when the acute seroconversion stage ends. HIV infection affects everybody differently, and many people experience few symptoms for the first 5 to 10 years of HIV infection.

How common are swollen lymph glands during HIV infection, and how long do they usually last?

It is common for people with HIV infection to have enlarged lymph nodes or swollen glands. This condition is called *progressive generalized lymphadenopathy* or *lymphadenopathy syndrome*. When swollen lymph nodes do occur, they are almost always detectable under the skin by touch. Figure 2.2 shows the areas of the body where swollen lymph nodes are most likely. Two thirds of people infected with HIV who have swollen lymph nodes experience them in their armpits, neck, head, and groin. Many people with HIV infection do not, however, experience long bouts of lymphadenopathy, and the presence of swollen lymph nodes does not signal the presence of full-blown AIDS. Swollen lymph nodes do not indicate how depleted the immune system

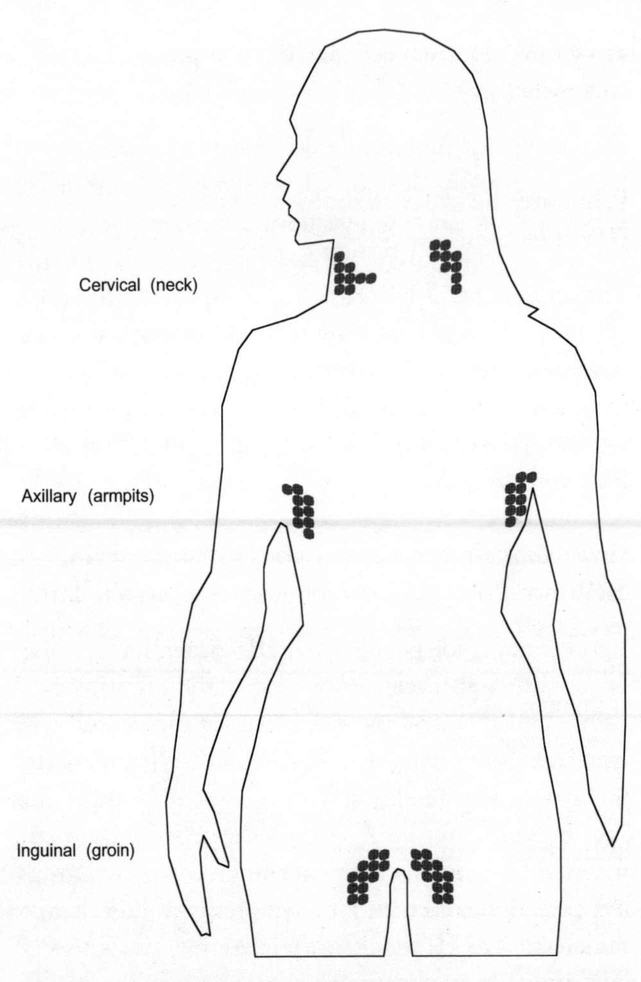

FIGURE 2.2. Lymph nodes that are most likely to be swollen during HIV lymphadenopathy.

may be. When lymphadenopathy does occur, it usually comes before most other symptoms of HIV infection and typically lasts a few months or longer.

What are the most common symptoms of HIV infection?

The most common symptoms of HIV infection are chronic low-grade fever, persistent fatigue, diarrhea, rashes or other skin conditions, unintentional weight loss of at least 10 pounds, night sweats, and thrush (an infection of the mouth or throat). These symptoms were once referred to as *AIDS-related complex (ARC)* because they were thought to always precede AIDS. However, the term ARC is no longer used because these symptoms do not mean that a person is about to get AIDS. Because HIV symptoms occur after the immune system has been run down, they can be accompanied by infections caused by bacteria, other viruses, fungi, and parasites.

Can symptoms of HIV infection occur in individuals who are not HIV positive?

If a person experiences true symptoms of HIV, he or she clearly has HIV infection. However, symptoms of HIV infection can resemble other illnesses, including the flu, mononucleosis, depression, and chronic fatigue syndrome. The only way to know whether a person has HIV infection is to perform an HIV antibody test. However, a person can continue to believe that their symptoms are from HIV infection even after repeatedly testing negative for HIV. Healthy people who become overly concerned about HIV infection are referred to as the *worried well* and can become preoccupied with believing they have HIV despite medical tests that show that they do not.

How do the symptoms of HIV differ from the symptoms of other sexually transmitted diseases?

Several infections are transmitted from person to person through sexual contact. Each sexually transmitted disease (STD) has its own cause, its own symptoms, and treatments. Unlike most other STDs, HIV can be transmitted through any contact with infected blood and does not cause an infection of the genital area itself. HIV does not cause burning, itching, open sores, or discharges. Syphilis, gonorrhea, genital warts, herpes simplex virus, and chlamydia are the most common STDs. These infections should not be confused with HIV infection—their causes and symptoms are completely different. But because HIV can be spread during sexual intimacy, it, too, is an STD. It is common for people to get more than one STD, so a person with HIV may have other STDs. People whose immune systems have been damaged by HIV infection may have worse cases of other sexually transmitted infections because they are unable to fight infections. Exhibit 2.2 lists common STDs and their symptoms and Appendix C provides a more detailed description of them.

EXHIBIT 2.2. STDs and Their Symptoms

STD	*Symptoms*
Chlamydia	7 to 28 days after infection Genital discharge, burning or painful urination, an urgent need to urinate, fever (men: swollen or tender testicles)
Gonorrhea	2 to 21 days after infection Thick yellow or white genital discharge, burning or painful urination, an urgent need to urinate (women: pain or cramps in lower abdomen)
Genital warts	1 to 18 months after infection Small bumpy warts on genital or anus, itching, burning
Hepatitis B	1 to 9 months after infection Flu symptoms, fatigue, yellowish skin (jaundice), dark urine, light-colored bowel movements
Herpes	1 to 30 days after infection Flulike symptoms, small painful blisters on genitals or mouth, itching or burning before blisters
Syphilis	3 to 12 weeks after infection Stage 1: Painless reddish-brown sore on genitals, mouth, breasts, or fingers lasting 1 to 5 weeks 1 to 6 months after infection Stage 2: Body rash, flu symptoms
Vaginal trichomoniasis (Trich)	Vaginal itching and burning, abnormal vaginal discharge

Is diarrhea a common symptom of HIV infection?

Yes. More than half of people with HIV infection experience serious bouts of diarrhea. There are, however, many causes of diarrhea in people with HIV infection, including medication side-effects and other viruses, bacteria, and parasites that infect the intestines after the immune system is damaged. Diarrhea itself can become life threatening, especially when it is a symptom of some AIDS-related illnesses. HIV infection of the small intestines can cause chronic diarrhea and can result in significant weight loss.

What does a skin rash from HIV infection look like?

People with HIV infection do not experience a single type of skin problem associated with HIV infection. A majority of people with HIV infection experience skin conditions that can be caused by bacteria, viruses, fungi, parasites, and cancers, as well as medication side effects. A rash caused by HIV itself often appears as small, raised reddish blotches on the face, upper body, arms, or legs.

AIDS

People generally think that those with HIV infection have AIDS because they often do not differentiate between HIV infection—being HIV positive—and having AIDS. In fact, only after HIV has depleted the body's defenses, a process that usually takes several years, does a person develop AIDS.

What is AIDS?

AIDS is the end stage of HIV infection. The letters *AIDS* stand for *acquired immune deficiency syndrome*:

- AIDS is an acquired disease. It is not inherited and it does not just develop on its own. The cause of AIDS is HIV, which is contracted from a source outside the body.
- AIDS is an immune disease because HIV damages the body's disease-fighting system.
- AIDS results from a deficiency in the immune system's cells caused by HIV, which leaves the body defenseless against diseases.
- AIDS is a syndrome, a group of symptoms and illnesses, rather than a single disease.

Does HIV always lead to AIDS?

To the best of our knowledge, most HIV-infected people eventually develop AIDS and ultimately die of AIDS-related illnesses. However, some people who were diagnosed with HIV during the first years of the AIDS epidemic in the United States felt healthy well into the new millennium. The strain of HIV that a person contracts seems important in determining the length of the disease. Advances in treatments for HIV infection and new medicines to prevent diseases associated with a depleted immune system also make it increasingly common for people who have not yet progressed to AIDS to live much longer without getting AIDS and for those with AIDS to survive longer. The time that a person can live with HIV infection without getting AIDS has increased considerably, and this trend is expected to continue.

At what point does a person have AIDS?

Several systems for diagnosing AIDS have been established. As more information about HIV infection and AIDS has become available, the diagnosis of AIDS has changed. The most common system for staging HIV infection comes from the Centers for Disease Control and Prevention (CDC). The first formal CDC AIDS diagnosis was proposed in 1982 and was based on a list of illnesses that people become vulnerable to when their immune system is depleted. The AIDS diagnosis was updated in 1985 and again in 1987 to include additional diseases. The 1987 definition of AIDS listed 23 diseases that occur when the immune system is badly damaged. The AIDS definition was once again expanded in 1993 to include 26 diseases and a diagnosis of AIDS based on damage to the immune system itself. Today people with HIV infection can be diagnosed with AIDS because they become ill with an HIV-related disease or because their immune system has sustained substantial damage (fewer than 200 T-helper cells per unit of blood) even if they have not yet become ill.

Is blurred vision a part of AIDS?

Not specifically. However, eye infections that can cause vision problems can occur when the immune system is damaged. The most common eye infection among AIDS patients is caused by cytomegalovirus (CMV). CMV can infect the retina (CMV retinitis) when T-helper lymphocytes are seriously depleted, usually when T-cell counts drop below 50 cells per unit of blood. The symptoms of CMV retinitis include loss in visual acuity, seeing floaters or images drift past the eye, and a reduction in peripheral vision. The damage caused by CMV to the retina is often irreparable, but the progression of the infection can usually be controlled with medications.

Are memory problems a sign of AIDS?

Cells that support, protect, and nurture primary brain cells have CD4 receptor sites on their surface and, like T-helper cells, are susceptible to HIV infection. HIV can enter the nervous system shortly after a person becomes HIV infected. HIV-infected nervous system cells produce chemicals that interfere with brain functions. People with advanced HIV infection and AIDS may experience a sense of sluggishness in their thinking and lapses in memory. However, it is less common for people with AIDS to suffer severe loss of memory and mental disabilities. It is also possible for memory problems to result from HIV-related opportunistic illnesses of the brain, such as toxoplasmosis or lymphoma, and from some medications used to treat HIV infection and its complications. Difficulties with concentration, attention, and memory can also be part of depression or anxiety. Thus, people with AIDS may experience memory slips, but these problems can have many causes, only one of which is HIV.

What are the first signs of AIDS?

AIDS is a process, not an event. There are no exact signs that predict when a person will get AIDS. In general, AIDS develops after the immune system declines to a point that the body cannot protect itself from disease. After the number of T-helper lymphocytes drops below 200 cells per unit of blood, a person is diagnosed with AIDS. For many people with HIV infection, their first AIDS illness is *Pneumocystis carinii pneumonia* (PCP). This is because most people already carry PCP and because symptoms can appear with only moderate damage to the immune system. However, medications are available that effectively prevent and treat PCP.

Why does the medical definition of AIDS keep changing?

Many things about the AIDS epidemic are constantly changing. With every new scientific discovery comes new information that changes how doctors treat HIV infection. Advances in knowledge also change the manner in which AIDS is viewed and how it is diagnosed. Classification systems are simplified and can often change to reflect new medical standards. New AIDS definitions can also address limitations of old diagnoses. For example, as more women became infected with HIV, AIDS diagnoses have changed to include diseases related to HIV infection in women.

What are AIDS-related illnesses?

People with severe damage to their immune system can develop many different infections and cancers. The illnesses that make up AIDS are rarely seen in people with healthy immune systems. These diseases take hold because of the body's inability to defend against them. AIDS-related illnesses are called *opportunistic illnesses* because they appear as a result of opportunity. Exhibit 2.3 lists the most typical AIDS-defining conditions, and Figure 2.3 shows the percentage of initial AIDS-defining opportunistic illnesses diagnosed in people with AIDS. See Appendix D for a more detailed description of the AIDS-related opportunistic illness.

How is AIDS related to tuberculosis (TB)?

TB was once well under control but has again come back with a vengeance to threaten global health. TB is a bacterial infection that primarily involves the lungs but can spread throughout the body. Mycobacterial TB is highly contagious; it is transmitted person to person by coughing or sneezing. TB can remain inac-

EXHIBIT 2.3. AIDS-Defining Conditions, 1993 Revision

- Candidiasis infection of bronchi, trachea, or lungs
- Candidiasis infection of esophagus
- Invasive cervical cancer
- Coccidioidomycosis, disseminated or extrapulmonary
- Cryptococcosis, extrapulmonary
- Cryptosporidiosis, intestinal, > 1 month
- Cytomegalovirus retinitis with loss of vision
- Cytomegalovirus disease
- HIV-related encephalopathy
- Herpes simplex infection, > 1 month
- Histoplasmosis, disseminated or extrapulmonary
- Isosporiasis, intestinal, > 1 month
- Kaposi's sarcoma
- Burkitt's lymphoma
- Immunoblastic lymphoma
- Primary lymphoma of brain
- *Mycobacterium avium complex*
- *Mycobacterium tuberculosis*
- *Myobacterium*, disseminated or extrapulmonary
- *Pneumocystis carinii pneumonia*
- Recurrent pneumonia
- Progressive multifocal leukoencephalopathy
- Recurrent salmonella septicemia
- Toxoplasmosis of the brain
- HIV wasting syndrome

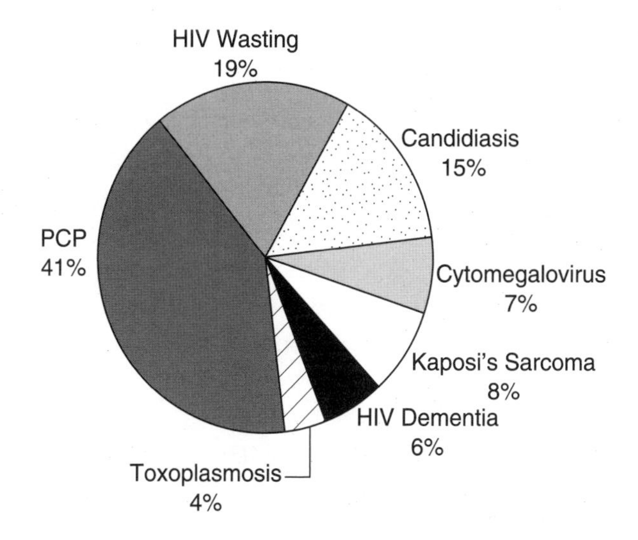

FIGURE 2.3. Percentages of initial AIDS-defining illnesses in people diagnosed with AIDS (CDC, 2001).

tive inside the body for a long time without causing symptoms and without being transmittable to others. TB is more likely to become active when the immune system is run down. In addition, TB is more difficult to treat when a person has advanced HIV infection because his or her body cannot assist in the fight against the infection.

Can a person not have any symptoms but still have AIDS?

Yes. It was once necessary to have at least one serious illness resulting from a severely impaired immune system before a person could be diagnosed with AIDS. However, today a diagnosis of AIDS is based strictly on the extent of immune system damage, regardless of whether the individual becomes ill. As noted earlier, a person whose blood test shows that they have less than 200 T-helper cells per milliliter of blood can be diagnosed with AIDS without ever experiencing a serious illness. AIDS-related illnesses are also often effectively treated, so a person with AIDS is not always ill.

How long can someone with AIDS expect to live?

AIDS progresses differently for every person. People can live 15 or 20 years after getting HIV without getting AIDS. Many individuals with AIDS can still live a long time, as many as 10 years after being diagnosed with AIDS. One factor that determines how long a person lives with HIV is what AIDS-related illnesses they contract. People first diagnosed with Kaposi's sarcoma, for example, are more likely to live longer than people diagnosed with PCP, who in turn survive longer than those initially diagnosed with other AIDS illnesses. Also important is how seriously the immune system is damaged when the illness occurs. However, the single most important factor in determining how long a person with HIV lives is their access to effective HIV treatment and medication that prevent opportunistic illnesses. Figure 2.4 shows the reduction in numbers of people dying from AIDS-

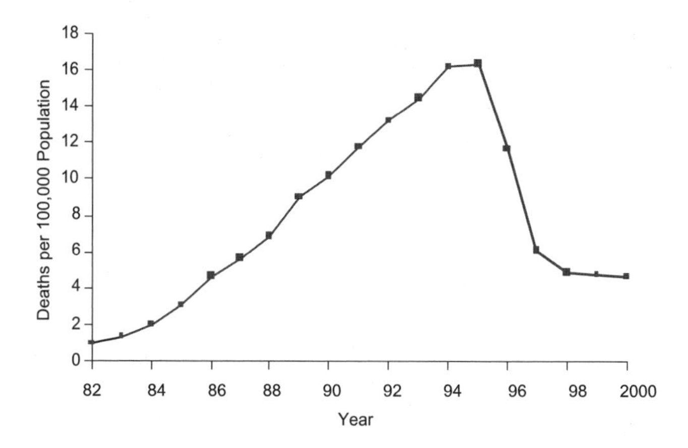

FIGURE 2.4. AIDS-related deaths in the United States, 1982–2000 (CDC, 2001).

related illnesses over the course of the HIV epidemic. The dramatic decrease in AIDS deaths is most likely the result of improved HIV treatment. The dramatic decline in deaths from AIDS that has occurred over the past several years is not seen in any other of the major causes of deaths in the United States (see Figure 2.5).

What are the "final stages" of AIDS?

The final stages of any terminal illness refer to the time when death is near. With respect to AIDS, the final stages are when the immune system is severely disabled and cannot respond to an illness that has become progressive and nonresponsive to treatment.

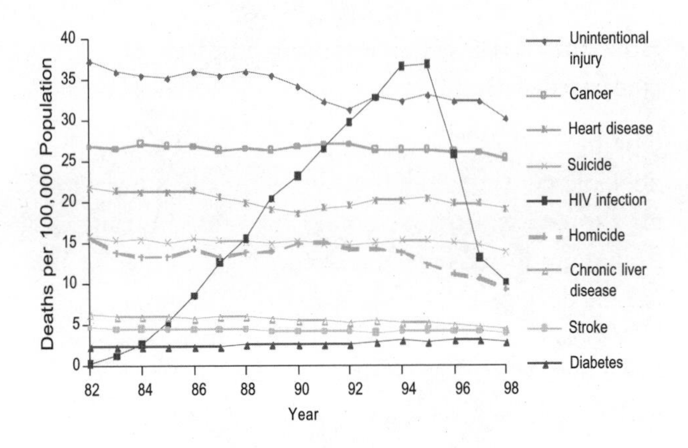

FIGURE 2.5. Changes in major causes of death in the United States between 1982 and 1998 (CDC, 2001).

Children With HIV and AIDS

HIV affects children in the same way it does adults—it infects T-helper lymphocyte cells and ultimately destroys the immune system. However, because young children do not have fully developed immune systems, HIV poses some additional problems. Most infected children get HIV from an HIV-positive mother during pregnancy or delivery. In the United States, 8,800 children younger than age 13 have been diagnosed with AIDS as of June 2000. The number has steadily decreased because of effective methods for preventing the transmission of HIV from mother to baby.

How does AIDS differ in young children as compared with adults?

Children with HIV infection live a shorter time than do adolescents and adults. Although babies born with HIV infection are not necessarily noticeably different from noninfected babies at birth, HIV-positive infants usually develop related illnesses within their first year. HIV-positive infants are also more likely than adults to suffer serious neurological disorders. Children infected with HIV also develop PCP and other lung diseases at earlier stages than do adults. Although the underlying destruction that HIV causes is the same in adults and children, the immature immune system of children seems to speed up the disease process.

How do doctors know when a baby has HIV infection?

An HIV antibody test alone is not enough to diagnose HIV infection in newborn babies because the mother's own antibodies cross over the placenta into the fetal bloodstream during pregnancy. Almost all babies born to HIV-positive women at first test HIV positive, even though less than half are actually infected. The test, therefore, detects the mother's antibodies in the newborn's blood. However, within 3 to 6 months after birth, the mother's antibodies dissipate from the baby's bloodstream. Babies who are actually infected with HIV begin to produce their own antibodies. HIV antibody tests in the first year of life do not, therefore, provide reliable information about whether a baby is infected. There are, however, more specialized tests that do provide information about whether a baby has been infected. A common test for directly detecting HIV is a PCR, like PCR tests for viral load described previously. Because PCR is a direct test for HIV genetic material, it is very specific to the diagnosis of HIV. In general, if a baby is healthy and does not test positive on any of the available blood tests at around age 18 months, the child is almost certainly not infected with HIV.

What are the symptoms of AIDS in children?

The symptoms of AIDS in children overlap with those of adults, but there are special considerations for diagnosing children with AIDS. Infants with AIDS are likely to have frequent and recurrent infections. Failure to thrive (i.e., stunted growth and development) is also a common problem. Babies with HIV infection are generally very sick, often suffering multiple infections. Children with AIDS are also likely to have serious infections and illnesses that affect the brain and nervous system.

Can children with AIDS get routine vaccinations and immunization?

Health authorities have recommended that children with HIV infection should be immunized on their usual schedule. Immunizations for HIV-positive babies are considered particularly important to help protect them from what could be a deadly infection. Pediatricians may have to adjust the particular types of vaccine used, but it may be more dangerous for children with HIV infection not to get immunized than to be immunized.

Summary

Like any other terminal illness, AIDS brings multiple losses and causes a person to go through many changes. However, AIDS is also different from almost all other life-threatening diseases. AIDS afflicts people of all ages, including infants and young adults; it does not have a cure; and it threatens the lives of more people each year. Also, because most people get HIV by injecting drugs or by having unsafe sex with an infected partner, there are many negative attitudes and stereotypes about people with HIV. The relationships among sex, drugs, and AIDS raise many questions answered in the next chapter.

3

How Does a Person Get HIV?

Most people know that HIV is spread through sexual intercourse and sharing needles to inject drugs. However, it remains unclear why certain sexual behaviors pose high risk for HIV infection, whereas other behaviors pose very low or no risk. Understanding how HIV is transmitted can empower people to protect themselves and their sex partners. Questions about HIV risks often stem from personal experience and concerns about one's own risks. Answering questions about HIV and AIDS requires talking openly about sex and drugs, topics that people often feel uncomfortable discussing. The reality of AIDS challenges us to be candid about sex and drugs and to ask explicit questions. Exhibit 3.1 summarizes the major risk behaviors for HIV, which form the basis for most questions about HIV transmission. Figures 3.1a and 3.1b show the percentages of men and women who have been infected with HIV by the various modes of transmission.

Anal Intercourse

Anal intercourse refers to sexual penetration in which the penis enters the anal–rectal cavity. Anal intercourse has caused almost all HIV infections among gay men because many, although by no means all, gay men practice anal intercourse. It is the behavior—anal intercourse—rather than being gay that creates risk for HIV, so anal intercourse between men and women poses just as much risk for HIV transmission when one of the partners has HIV.

What makes anal intercourse so risky for HIV infection?

Anal intercourse with an HIV-positive partner and without the protection of latex condoms carries greater risk for HIV infection than any other sexual act. Several factors make anal intercourse a risky behavior:

- The walls of the anus and rectum are thin and richly supplied with blood vessels, making tears or scratches common during sexual penetration.
- The anal opening is narrow and constricts when stimulated, increasing the chances for trauma and bleeding.
- Direct access of HIV-infected semen to the bloodstream and lymph nodes occurs easily when rectal walls are damaged.
- Torn tissues in the rectum can expose the mucous membranes of the penis to HIV-infected blood, creating risk for both partners.

EXHIBIT 3.1. Risk Behaviors for HIV and Other STDs

Behavior	*Risk*
Anal intercourse	Highest risk sexual behavior Accounts for vast majority of HIV infections in gay and bisexual men
Vaginal intercourse	Very high-risk behavior Accounts for most HIV infections in the world
Oral–genital contact	Uncertain risk for HIV infection High risk for transmission of herpes, gonorrhea, syphilis, and other STDs
Kissing	No known risks for HIV transmission in the absence of blood

Even when there are no tears in the rectal lining, anal intercourse poses high risk for HIV infection because M-cells and Langerhans cells, which transport foreign material to the immune system to protect against infection, are located in the mucous lining and may be infected. In the case of HIV, however, M-cells and Langerhans cells transport the virus to immune cells that are vulnerable to HIV infection.

Can anal intercourse be made more or less risky?

The risk posed by anal intercourse increases when there is trauma or injury to the walls of the rectum. Research shows that scratches or tears to mucous mem-

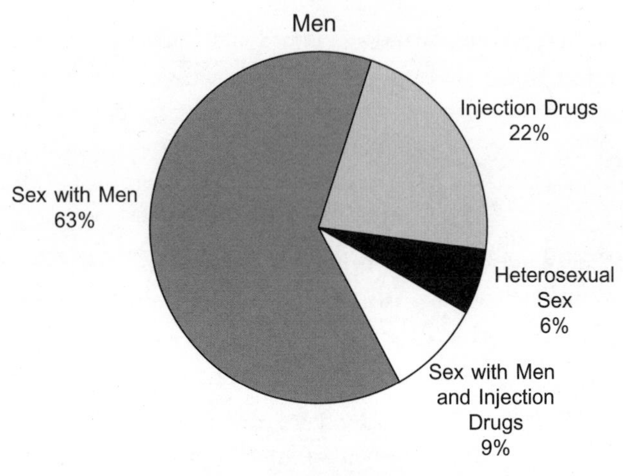

A

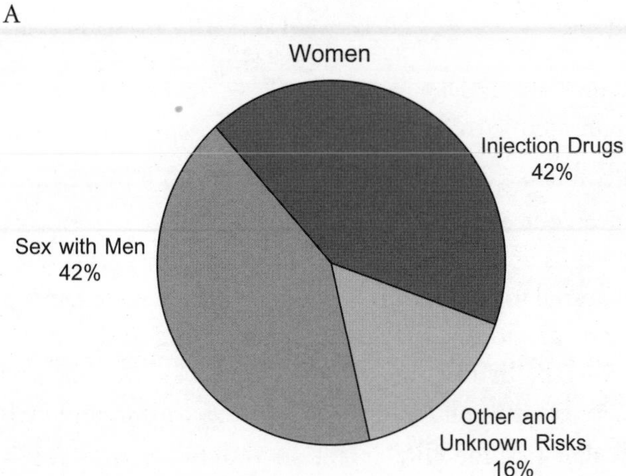

B

FIGURES 3.1A–B. Percentages of men and women in the United States who contracted HIV through various modes of transmission.

branes make anal intercourse twice as risky for HIV infection as anal intercourse in the absence of lacerations. Another factor that increases the risk is the stage of HIV infection present when a person engages in unprotected anal intercourse. Because there is an abundance of virus in the bloodstream during the earliest periods of HIV infection, risk may be greatest when individuals are least likely to know that they are HIV positive. Risk is also higher at the later stages of HIV infection, when the disease has progressed to AIDS and levels of HIV in the blood are again high. Risk for HIV infection also increases with the number of anal intercourse partners. For example, gay men with five partners with whom they engage in anal intercourse are at 18 times greater risk for HIV infection than men with only one unprotected anal intercourse partner. The more unsafe partners a person has, the higher the odds are that one of the partners is HIV positive. The best way to make anal intercourse less risky is to use latex condoms.

Can a man get HIV from anal intercourse if he is the one who puts his penis in his partner?

Sexual risk for HIV infection is a two-way street—both partners are at risk. A man who inserts his penis into an HIV-positive partner during anal intercourse is at risk for HIV infection. Without the protection of a latex condom, the skin covering the penis and the mucous membranes of the urethral opening are exposed to the lining of the rectum, which, as described earlier, is likely to bleed during anal intercourse. Small scratches can occur on the penis during intercourse, providing another port of entry for the virus into the bloodstream. However, little cuts or scratches are not even necessary for HIV transmission to occur. Like the walls of the rectum, the mucous membranes of the urethra are rich with cells that transport foreign material to the immune system for elimination. HIV binds to these cells, which then carry the virus to vulnerable immune system cells.

Is it riskier if a partner is the one who receives a man's penis during anal intercourse?

Yes. During anal intercourse the receptive partner is at considerably higher risk for HIV infection. This is because of the large amount of HIV that can exist in semen. Risk for HIV infection is at least twice as great for the receiving partner compared with the inserting partner during anal intercourse.

Can a man get HIV if he has anal intercourse with a woman?

Yes. It is a mistake to think that only homosexual men have anal intercourse. About one in five young heterosexual couples practice anal intercourse. Anal intercourse is sometimes practiced as a means of avoiding pregnancy, to maintain "virginity," or as a preference. For the same reasons that anal intercourse poses high risk for two men who have sex, anal intercourse between men and women carries high risk as well.

Can a person get HIV if he or she had anal intercourse just one time?

Yes. A person can get HIV infection from just one anal intercourse experience with an HIV-positive partner. Of course, some people have had many anal intercourse experiences with an infected partner and have not gotten infected, whereas others have been infected after having anal intercourse a single time. No one knows exactly why some people get infected faster than others, but the chance of infection is present each time a person has intercourse with an HIV-infected partner without using a condom.

Does HIV get transmitted during anal intercourse even if there is no ejaculation?

HIV is present in the mucous membranes and blood of an HIV-infected person. A man who inserts his penis into the anus of an HIV-infected male or female sex partner is at risk regardless of whether he ejaculates. For the receiving partner, either male or female, the greater the amount of fluid that enters the rectum, the more HIV will be present, increasing the chances for infection. However, even if the penis is withdrawn before ejaculation, there is still some risk for HIV transmission because the fluids that come out of the tip of the penis before ejaculation contain HIV.

Vaginal Intercourse

The majority of people in the world who have AIDS became HIV infected through vaginal intercourse. Regardless of whether a person is originally infected with HIV from sex, injecting drugs, or a blood transfusion, a man or woman can infect their sexual partners during vaginal intercourse.

Can a man get HIV from a woman?

Yes. Men get HIV from having vaginal intercourse with HIV-positive women. Although in North America most men have gotten HIV from sex with other men or from injecting drugs, many men have gotten HIV from vaginal intercourse. Throughout the world, most men with AIDS became HIV infected through vaginal intercourse.

How do men get HIV from vaginal intercourse?

Fluids from the mucous lining of an HIV-positive woman's vagina contain a sufficient amount of virus to cause infection. HIV can enter the man's body through the urinary opening at the tip of his penis or through small scratches on his penis. Microscopic cuts or tears in the skin allow HIV to enter the body. Sores, blisters, or ulcers caused by other sexually transmitted diseases (STDs) such as gonorrhea, genital herpes, and syphilis make it especially easy for HIV to enter the body.

Can a woman get HIV from a man?

Yes. Most women who have AIDS were infected with HIV from having vaginal intercourse with an HIV-positive man. Forty percent of all women in the United States who have AIDS became HIV infected from intercourse with a man who had sex with other men, injected drugs, or had sex with an infected woman.

How do women get HIV from vaginal intercourse?

During vaginal intercourse an HIV-positive man deposits infected semen into the vagina, exposing the vagina to HIV. Once the semen is in the vagina, there are many ways that HIV enters the bloodstream. The vaginal walls are covered by a mucous lining that covers a rich supply of blood vessels, allowing HIV to access the bloodstream through small scratches on the surface of the vaginal lining. Vaginal mucous membranes also contain a rich supply of infectable immune cells. Research has shown that HIV is actually absorbed by the vaginal mucous lining even when there are no apparent openings. Small scratches do, however, make it easier for HIV to enter the bloodstream, and therefore increase the risk for HIV infection. Cuts or abrasions in the vagina, especially sores caused by infections, including sexually transmitted infections, increase the rate of HIV transmission during vaginal intercourse.

Is there still risk if the penis is pulled out of the vagina before ejaculation?

Yes. For a person to get HIV there must be a sufficient amount of virus present to enter the body. Interrupting intercourse by withdrawing the penis from the vagina before ejaculation results in less exposure to infected fluids, both vaginal fluids exposed to the penis and ejaculation fluids exposed to the vagina. However, withdrawal does not necessarily prevent HIV transmission. Vaginal fluids come in contact with the penis during intercourse whether or not the penis is withdrawn before ejaculation. Also, the fluids that precede ejaculation can contain sufficient amounts of HIV to cause infection. Withdrawal before ejaculation may reduce risk, but it cannot completely protect people from HIV.

Does vaginal intercourse during a woman's period increase the risk of HIV infection?

Sex during the time that a woman is menstruating can increase the chances of transmitting HIV from an infected woman to her sex partner because of the presence of blood. The greatest amount of HIV is found in infected blood, which could increase the amount of virus a partner is exposed to when having sex during the menstrual period.

Who is at greater risk for getting HIV during vaginal intercourse, the man or the woman?

HIV enters the bloodstream when a sufficient amount of virus is exposed to mucous linings or has another point of entry into the body. HIV exists in fluids and mucous membranes that line the vagina, so men are at risk for HIV infection during vaginal intercourse. However, because semen can carry a very high dose of HIV and because the mucous lining of the vagina provides a large surface area for HIV transmission, there is a greater risk for HIV infection from an infected man to an uninfected woman. HIV transmission from men to women during vaginal intercourse can be 2 to 10 times as likely when compared with risk for infection from women to men. Unfortunately, some men have taken this to mean that they are at low risk for HIV infection when they have sex with an infected woman. This belief is false, however, because even though the risk may be lower for men than women, it does not mean that men are at low risk.

Oral Sex

Sexual contact where one partner uses the mouth to stimulate the partner's genitals is practiced by as many as 80% of adults in sexual relationships. Oral sex has been the most controversial mode of possible HIV transmission. Of all of the calls received by AIDS information hotlines asking about behaviors that put people at risk for HIV, the most common questions concern oral sex.

What STDs can a person get from oral sex?

The majority of STDs occur when infected mucous membranes come in contact with uninfected mucous membranes. Herpes simplex virus, gonorrhea, and syphilis infections of the lips, mouth, or throat can cause infection of the genitals, and vice versa.

How many people have been infected with HIV through oral sex?

It is impossible to know. People who engage in oral sex also often have vaginal or anal sex. Researchers have tried to examine the risk for HIV infection from oral sex by studying the past sexual behaviors of people who have become infected. These studies show that far fewer people have been infected with HIV from oral sex alone than from anal or vaginal intercourse. However, sexual contact that involves taking vaginal fluids or semen into the mouth must be considered to pose some risk for HIV infection because a small number of people seem to have been infected through oral–genital contact.

Does saliva destroy HIV and make oral sex safe?

No. Enzymes and other chemicals in saliva do inactivate HIV. The envelope that surrounds the HIV core is fragile and easily damaged by substances found in saliva. However, HIV remains protected inside infected immune cells of the oral mucous lining. The best way to decrease the possibility of HIV transmission during oral sex is to use a latex condom or other barrier, or to completely avoid getting semen or vaginal fluids in the mouth.

Is one type of oral sex riskier for HIV than another?

There are two types of oral–genital sex:

- *Fellatio:* mouth-to-penis sex where a man's penis is stimulated by his partner's mouth and lips.
- *Cunnilingus:* mouth-to-vagina sex where a woman's genitals are stimulated by her partner.

The risks for HIV from all four types of oral sex (giving or receiving fellatio or cunnilingus) are lower than anal and vaginal intercourse. It appears that the riskiest kind of oral sex is when a man or woman performs fellatio on a man who has HIV, getting semen in the mouth. This act involves the greatest amount of exposure of the oral mucous membranes to HIV. Cunnilingus appears to carry less risk for HIV infection than does fellatio.

Can a person get HIV from sex that involves mouth-to-breast contact?

Unless there are open sores or cracked nipples or the woman is producing breast milk (lactating), mouth-to-breast stimulation does not place a person at risk for giving or getting HIV.

What can make oral sex riskier for HIV infection?

Just like vaginal and anal intercourse, the risk of getting or giving HIV during oral sex increases when there are cuts, sores, or other lesions in the mouth, which allow easier access of HIV to the bloodstream. Trauma that can result from "rough oral sex" would also likely increase risk for HIV transmission. Cold sores, gum diseases, canker sores, or minor cuts in the mouth can contain infection-fighting immune cells that are vulnerable to HIV infection. Although there is no evidence that cuts or sores in the mouth are necessary for HIV infection to occur, they would surely increase HIV's access to infectable cells.

If a person has oral sex, wouldn't the stomach acids kill HIV, making oral sex safe?

Stomach acids are strong and immediately inactivate HIV. However, it is a myth that HIV infection happens as a result of swallowing vaginal fluids or semen. Instead, the risk for HIV infection during oral sex is from HIV being absorbed by the mucous membranes of the mouth and throat or through a sore or other lesions in or around the mouth.

How risky is oral–anal (mouth-to-anus) sex?

Oral-anal sex, sometimes called *rimming*, does not appear to carry high risk for HIV infection unless there is blood present. However, oral–anal sex is a high-risk behavior for a number of other serious diseases, including hepatitis B virus, herpes simplex virus, cytomegalovirus, and various parasites.

Is it possible to have oral sex that is completely safe?

It is entirely possible for oral–genital contact to be free of any risk for HIV transmission. The risk for oral–genital transmission of HIV is low. Sexual contact without the transfer of fluids from the vagina or the penis to the mouth, and vice versa, poses no risk for HIV infection—assuming that there are no open sores on the mouth or genitals. Sexual stimulation without ejaculation and avoidance of contact with pre-ejaculation fluids makes fellatio as safe as any other type of contact between skin and mucous membranes. The same is true for stimulation of the female genitals without contacting vaginal fluids. An alternative way to make oral sex virtually risk free is to use latex barriers. Condoms can nearly eliminate the risk for HIV infection during fellatio. Similarly, proper use of small sheets of latex, such as dental dams or nonporous plastic wraps, eliminates contact with vaginal fluids and removes the risk of HIV infection.

Kissing

Kissing is perhaps second only to hugging as the most frequent form of intimate contact. Many viruses are spread through kissing, such as those that cause colds, flu, and infectious mononucleosis ("the kissing disease"). Concerns that HIV transmission occurs during deep kissing is understandable but not supported by the facts.

Can a person get AIDS from deep kissing?

There is one documented case of a woman who apparently became infected with HIV as a result of deep kissing. In this case, the man reported having had bleeding gums shortly before kissing. The unlikelihood of infection by kissing can be explained by the tiny amount of HIV in saliva and the presence of chemicals and enzymes in saliva that damage HIV's protective envelope. Kissing in the absence of blood is therefore a safe behavior.

If a person passionately kisses someone who has mouth sores, could that person be at risk?

It is theoretically possible to get HIV from kissing a person who has HIV and has open sores in or around the mouth or blood in the saliva. Even in these cases, however, the chances for HIV infection seem remote; for all practical purposes, kissing does not pose a risk for HIV infection.

Other Aspects of Sex

Sexual relationships are complex and involve more than specific sex acts. Questions regarding sex and AIDS often pertain to many of the complexities of intimate relationships.

How often do people with HIV have sex without telling their partners that they are infected?

Individuals with HIV infection have the responsibility of telling their sex partners about their HIV status before having sex. Disclosure involves risking rejection, so each individual handles this situation differently. Some people choose not to engage in sex at all after they have tested HIV positive. Others tell people they are intimate with about their HIV status right away. However, some people with HIV choose to practice only safe sex and not tell their partners they have HIV. When a person's HIV status is shared, it allows a couple to decide how best to protect each other. Research has shown that a minority of people with HIV do not tell their casual sex partners that they have HIV, but most individuals do tell their regular, or main, partners.

If two people both have HIV, are there concerns about them having unprotected sex?

Yes. A major barrier to sexual relations, namely the risk of spreading HIV, is removed when both people know they are already HIV positive. However, there are health concerns for HIV-positive couples who choose to have unsafe sex with each other. Co-infection with other diseases, particularly other sexually transmitted viruses, bacteria, and parasites, poses serious health risks for people with HIV. Introducing a new infection can stimulate and activate HIV to begin replicating itself. Co-infections can also cause illnesses that are especially difficult to treat in people with suppressed immune systems. Because there are many strains of HIV and some are more virulent than others, becoming reinfected with HIV may be a health hazard. Transmission of HIV-treatment-resistant strains of virus may also occur between partners. These potential risks raise concerns about unprotected sex between HIV-positive partners.

Can a person get HIV by using "sex toys"?

HIV can remain on objects used during sex, such as vibrators or dildos, and so in theory it can be passed from one person to another. Because HIV cannot remain viable for long outside of the body, the risk of HIV transmission from objects is low. However, sex toys can cause small tears or scratches on the fragile vaginal and anal mucous linings, making the use of sex toys potentially risky. Using sex toys can be completely safe, however, under the following conditions:

- The toy is not shared; each person has his or her own.

- If they are shared, they must be cleaned between use by each person.
- Latex condoms are placed over sex toys, such as dildos, during their use and changed between uses by each partner.

Sharing Needles

Sharing needles and other drug injection equipment can be an intimate part of using drugs. Needle sharing occurs in an interpersonal relationship. Needle sharing may be a form of intimacy, but there are economic aspects as well. Because drug use is illegal, injection equipment is usually scarce. People who inject drugs can therefore be forced to use dirty needles and share injection equipment. For these reasons, sharing needles to inject drugs is a major factor in the spread of HIV/AIDS.

What makes sharing needles so risky for HIV?

To allow fluids to flow, injection needles are hollow, and both the inside and outside of the needles come in contact with blood. In addition, it is common for blood to be drawn into the syringe while injecting, contaminating the entire syringe apparatus—which includes a cotton, a corker, and a cooker, collectively referred to as *works*. Blood is present during injection when drugs are shot up into the bloodstream (intravenous drug use). HIV-infected blood can therefore be passed directly from the bloodstream of one person to that of another.

How long can a needle cause infection after it has been used?

It is not possible to know exactly how long HIV remains viable outside of the body. Research has shown that HIV does not survive indefinitely on surfaces under laboratory conditions. However, HIV in dried blood is capable of causing infection for several days. A thin film of dried blood containing HIV can be found in and on needles, as well as on plungers and syringes. Even a small amount of residual blood can cause HIV infection when it comes in contact with another person's bloodstream.

Can a person get HIV from injecting drugs if he or she uses clean needles?

No. Drugs and the needles used to inject drugs do not themselves cause HIV infection. A person who injects drugs is at risk for HIV infection only when the needle, syringe, or other equipment is contaminated by HIV-infected blood.

How can a person get clean needles to avoid HIV infection?

Until recently, the only way to get sterile injection equipment was with a doctor's prescription, which is not usually given for illicit drugs. So people have relied on an underground supply of used needles to inject. However, since it was first learned that dirty needles were fueling the AIDS epidemic, laws have been changed in some states to allow free access to clean needles and syringes. Some programs exchange used needles and syringes for clean ones. Studies have repeatedly shown that providing clean needles successfully prevents HIV infections.

If a person gets HIV from sharing needles, can he or she give it to a non-drug-using sex partner?

HIV infects immune cells and is passed through contact with HIV-infected blood and other body fluids regardless of how a person became infected. A person who was HIV infected by sharing needles can pass the virus on through any behaviors that expose people to infected body fluids. More than 16% of women with AIDS in the United States became HIV infected by having sex with a man who got HIV from injecting drugs, and this rate may be higher in other countries with emerging HIV epidemics among injection drug users.

Pregnancy and Childbirth

Pregnant women with HIV infection can pass the virus on to their fetuses and newborns. The majority of children with AIDS in the world have gotten HIV during pregnancy or the birth process.

If a pregnant woman has HIV, what are the chances that her baby will get infected?

Researchers cannot quantify the risk of HIV transmission during pregnancy or childbirth (or any other method of HIV transmission, for that matter). The rate of infection from mother to fetus is, however, very high because of the exposure to large amounts of blood. It is estimated that about one third of all babies born to untreated HIV-positive mothers get the virus during pregnancy or delivery. The risk of HIV transmission depends on factors such as the stage of HIV infection a mother is at—women who are at early and later stages of HIV infection are at higher risk for transmitting the virus to their babies. And whether a mother is receiving anti-HIV medications is also an important factor because treatments for HIV significantly reduce the risk of HIV transmission during pregnancy.

How is HIV transmitted from mother to child?

Babies born to HIV-positive mothers can get the virus in several ways. While in the womb, the fetus is protected by the placenta, which forms a barrier between the maternal and fetal bloodstreams. For infection to occur during pregnancy, it is necessary for the placenta itself to first become infected before the virus can be passed on to the fetus. Infection is also possible during labor and delivery, when large amounts of the mother's blood bathe the newborn during passage through the birth canal. Finally, a mother can infect her infant during breast-feeding because HIV is found in breast milk. Cracks in breast nipples can also allow the mother's blood to mix with her milk, further increasing the risk of infection.

Can a woman who gets HIV while she is pregnant give the virus to the fetus?

Yes. It does not take long for HIV to establish itself in the body. A woman who contracts HIV during her pregnancy can transmit the virus to her baby.

Playing the Odds

As a general rule, people want to feel safe. Some people try to predict events in their daily lives, carefully calculating the risks they are willing to take. Out of the desire to feel safe, people often underestimate the risk they are taking by behaviors they frequently practice, and they overestimate the risk of behaviors that they have rarely practiced. The concerns that people have about the risk of HIV infection can spawn many questions.

Is it possible to get HIV from having intercourse with a person you have been with for years?

Yes, it is possible to get HIV from having sexual intercourse with any person who is HIV infected. Many people have been infected with HIV from a person they love and whom they have been with for a long time. People often do not know they are at risk or that they are putting their loved ones at risk. Loved ones give us a sense of security. However, the HIV epidemic includes many individuals who unknowingly became infected by an HIV-positive partner they love.

Can a person get infected from a sex partner who has HIV but has an undetectable viral load?

Yes. A person who has an undetectable viral load can transmit HIV to sex partners. An undetectable viral load does not mean that a person no longer has the virus. In addition, there is only a weak association between viral load in blood (which the viral load test is based on) and viral load in semen and vaginal fluids. So a person with an undetectable viral load may in fact be infectious.

Are uncircumcised men at greater risk for getting HIV infection?

Uncircumcised men may be at higher risk for getting HIV infection when compared with circumcised men. Infections under the foreskin allow easy access to the bloodstream and infectable immune cells. Minor infections under the foreskin of an uncircumcised penis can harbor a multitude of infection-fighting immune cells; in an HIV-positive man, many of these cells are infected, which increases the risk of transmitting the virus to a partner.

Can a person get HIV the first time he or she has sexual intercourse?

Yes. Sexual intercourse with a person who has HIV without using latex condoms is all that it takes to get infected. It does not matter whether a person has ever had sex before. It is myth that only the sexually promiscuous become HIV infected. The risk of getting HIV increases with more frequent sexual encounters with a variety of partners, but it only takes one encounter with one infected person to become HIV infected. If a person has only one partner who is HIV infected, the risk of transmission accumulates over the course of that relationship.

How many times does a person have to have sex to be at risk for HIV infection?

A person can have sex many times with an HIV-positive partner and not get infected. On the other hand, a person can become HIV infected after having sex just once. It is impossible to know the exact odds of getting infected during any one sexual act for any given individual because so many factors increase and decrease risk.

Which sexual activities are considered the riskiest and the safest?

The risk of getting or giving HIV during any single sexual act is determined by the amount of HIV that

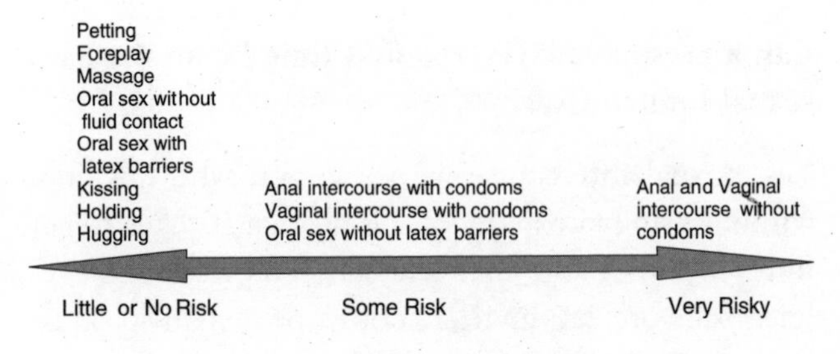

FIGURE 3.2. HIV risk behavior continuum.

enters another person's body and the virus's access to infectable cells. For example, anal intercourse is a high-risk activity for HIV infection because large amounts of virus are brought in contact with thin mucous membranes containing infectable cells and broken blood vessels. On the other hand, some behaviors, such as caressing or body rubbing, are virtually risk free because they do not involve exposure to bodily fluids. The highest risk of HIV transmission is presented by those behaviors that allow semen, vaginal fluids, or blood to enter another person's body. A middle level of risk exists for those acts where the virus could enter the body, such as intercourse with latex condoms, but it is to a significantly less degree than the high-risk category. Figure 3.2 illustrates the relative risks for HIV transmission along a continuum of behavioral risks.

Is it possible for HIV infection to occur during sex even when there are no cuts or tears on a person's genitals?

Yes. It is not necessary for cuts or tears to be present during sex for infection to occur because HIV is absorbed directly into mucous membranes. Cuts or tears on the skin or mucous membranes during sexual intercourse can facilitate the transmission of HIV because of greater access to the bloodstream. Openings in the skin or mucous membranes also allow direct contact with infected blood.

Can a person get HIV if his or her sex partner never injected drugs and this was a first sexual relationship?

Today, adults who have never injected drugs or had sexual intercourse are almost certainly not infected with HIV and cannot, therefore, infect their first sex partner. It is a person's history—what they have done—not who they are that creates risk for HIV/AIDS.

How can a person tell if a sex partner is infected with HIV?

The only way to know if a person has HIV infection is through a blood test. It is impossible for a person to know if someone has HIV by looking at that person. Knowing the past risk history of a sex partner can raise warning signals that the partner may be infected, but even people who seem to have been at low risk may have been infected with HIV.

Summary

The vast majority of HIV infections in the United States and the world result from either sexual intercourse with an infected partner or sharing injection equipment used to inject drugs. The fact that HIV is transmitted in only a few specific ways is one of the few bright spots in the AIDS epidemic. With only a few exceptions, a person has to actively do something to get the virus. Because the AIDS epidemic is fueled by common sexual risk behaviors, the virus has spread fastest in groups that practice these behaviors.

4

Who Is at Risk for AIDS?

There is not just one AIDS epidemic; rather, there are many AIDS epidemics, all unfolding at once. In the earlier days of AIDS, it was convenient to think of certain people as being at risk and not others. But as AIDS has spread and we have learned more about the specific behaviors that place people at risk, the notion of risk groups has become less meaningful. It is the things that people do that cause HIV infection, not who they are. Practicing high-risk behaviors in communities with high rates of HIV places people at greatest risk. Many questions remain about HIV risks within specific communities, particularly communities that have been most affected by AIDS. Exhibit 4.1 presents a personal risk assessment that can help individuals identify their own personal risk history.

Gay and Bisexual Men

Gay men (men who identify themselves as being sexually and affectionately attracted to other men) and

EXHIBIT 4.1. Personal Assessment of Risks for Sexually Transmitted Diseases

Risk factor	*Risk explanation*
How many sex partners have you ever had?	The more sex partners, the more risk.
How often do you drink alcohol or use drugs before having sex?	Substance use can reduce the likelihood of practicing safer sex.
When you have sex, how often do you use a condom?	Consistent use of condoms offers the best protection aside from abstinence.
Have you ever used needles to shoot drugs?	Each of these behaviors can increase the risk for HIV. The more risk factors in a person's history, the greater the risk.
Have you ever given or taken something to trade for sex, like money, drugs, or a place to stay?	
Have you ever had a sexual disease (STD)?	Other STDs are transmitted like HIV and can increase chances of HIV transmission.
Have you had a sex partner who you think shot up drugs?	A person who got HIV from shooting drugs can transmit the virus to sex partners.

continued

bisexual men (men who identify themselves as sexually and affectionately attracted to men and women) practice a wide variety of sexual behaviors. Regardless of a man's sexual orientation or sexual identity, men who

EXHIBIT 4.1. *Continued*

Risk factor	*Risk explanation*
Have you had a sex partner who you think had other sex partners?	Having other sex partners introduces risks for spreading infection.
Are you a man who has had anal sex with other men?	Anal sex is high risk for HIV, so men who practice anal sex with men are at high risk.
Have you had a sex partner who you think could have had HIV?	A partner must have HIV to transmit it to others.
Have you had a sex partner who you think could have had an STD?	Partners who have had STDs are at risk for HIV and therefore passing the virus to new partners.
Have you had sex with someone once and never seen them again?	Not knowing a partner's history makes you unaware of risks.

Note. The more risk factors a person endorses the greater their risk has been for HIV infection. Some risk factors may carry more risk than others and risk can depend on where and when the behaviors occurred.

have sex with men may be at risk for HIV infection. Of all of the sexual activities that men practice together, anal intercourse carries the greatest risk for HIV infection.

Is AIDS a "gay" disease?

No. Early in the U.S. AIDS epidemic, many people thought that there must be something specific about gay men and their lifestyle that was responsible for AIDS. In fact, the earliest name for AIDS was gay-related immune disorder. However, people believed that AIDS was a "gay" disease because they did not know about the devastating growth of AIDS among heterosexual men and women in Africa. It was easy to blame gay men for AIDS because it helped to psychologically distance the disease from the heterosexual population. We now know that thinking of AIDS as a gay disease was not only harmful to gay men but likely cost lives because of delayed prevention and education activities for the general public.

Why do so many gay men have AIDS?

Only a minority of people who have AIDS are men who got the virus from having sex with other men. However, the HIV epidemics in North America and Western Europe have shown a different pattern. The earliest cases of HIV infection in North America occurred in large cities among men who had anal intercourse with other men. The virus then spread rapidly within gay communities for several reasons:

- The virus became concentrated within the sexual networks of men who have sex with men.

- The practice of anal intercourse provided an efficient means for the virus to gain access to a sex partner's bloodstream.
- Nobody knew that HIV existed and that it was being spread.

HIV was passed from one man to another for years before the first case of AIDS and even longer before HIV was actually discovered, so gay men were quickly and unknowingly getting infected.

Is AIDS decreasing in gay communities?

The relative number of AIDS cases has been declining in gay communities, particularly in U.S. cities. For example, in 1989, 64% of men with AIDS had gotten HIV from homosexual sex, whereas in 1994 homosexual sex caused HIV infection in 53% of men with AIDS, and in 2000 this rate was down to 44%. The reason for the relative decline of AIDS in gay communities in the United States can be attributed to changes that gay men have made in their sexual practices and the rise in AIDS among other groups of people. From the beginning, grassroots organizations educated gay men about AIDS and how sexual relationships can be both meaningful and safe. The decline in AIDS cases reflects the care that gay men have had for themselves, their partners, and their communities. However, these education efforts have not been entirely successful at reaching all men who have sex with men. In particular, ethnic minority men who have sex with men have been the most difficult to reach and consequently have some of the highest rates of HIV infection.

Are teenagers who experiment with homosexuality at risk?

Adolescence is a time for self-discovery—not just sexual discovery, but complete self-discovery. Whether a person is gay, bisexual, straight, or unsure, the feelings and experiences that accompany sexual orientation emerge in adolescence. Young men who have sex with men are at extremely high risk of HIV infection if they have anal intercourse without condoms. In some cities, such as San Francisco and New York, there is great concern that young men are in the midst of a new wave of the AIDS epidemic.

Do men who have sex while in prison get HIV?

Yes. Men who have anal intercourse with other men while in prison are at high risk for HIV infection for several reasons:

- Many men are in prison for drug crimes, so many prisoners have injected drugs and may have been infected with HIV. These same prisoners may have sex with other inmates.
- Prisons often have underground networks of inmates who inject drugs, spreading the virus within prisons.

- Injecting drugs in prison involves sharing needles because it is not possible to get sterile injection equipment.
- Studies show that a large number of men have sex with other inmates while they are incarcerated, and men are often raped in prison.
- Because sex between men in prison is not permitted and usually constitutes a crime, there are usually no condoms available to inmates.
- The lack of condoms in prison can bring men to use other makeshift barriers, such as fingers cut from latex gloves, which can actually increase the risk of infection.
- Prisons have networks of inmates who engage in homosexual acts within which HIV can rapidly spread.

Thus, HIV infection is an epidemic in prisons, and men who leave prisons infected with HIV can spread the virus to others.

Lesbians and Bisexual Women

Sex between women, like sex between men, involves a great variety of behaviors. However, the behaviors that women engage in do not usually carry as high a risk of HIV infection because there are few opportunities for large amounts of the virus to gain access to a partner's bloodstream.

How many women have gotten HIV from having sex with other women?

Just like any other means of getting HIV, it is impossible to know how many women have gotten the virus from having sex with other women. However, it appears that very few women have been infected from having sex with other women. One early study of 960,000 women in the United States who donated blood did not find a single case of HIV infection among women who exclusively had sexual contact with other women. Another study of more than 1,000 women who were infected with HIV identified only one woman who reported sexual contact with other women as her only risk factor for HIV infection. However, many lesbians have been infected with HIV from either having sex with men or injecting drugs. Because vaginal fluids contain HIV, there is some risk of infection when two women are sexually intimate. However, it is male sex partners who have infected most women who contracted HIV through sexual behavior.

What can place a lesbian at high risk for HIV?

The sexual acts between women that carry high risk for transmitting HIV are cunnilingus, oral–vaginal contact, and sharing sex toys. However, the risk of HIV infection from cunnilingus appears small unless there are open cuts or sores in the mouth or on the vagina. Sexual practices that involve exposure to blood, such as rough sex or sex during menstruation, would also carry the highest risks for HIV.

Heterosexual Men and Women

Most of the people who have AIDS are heterosexual. Men and women who have vaginal intercourse without the protection of latex condoms are at risk of HIV infection, particularly when they do not know for sure that they or their partners are HIV negative.

Are heterosexual men and women really at risk?

Yes. Heterosexual people who practice vaginal or anal intercourse without condoms can be at risk for getting HIV. The number of people in the United States who become infected through vaginal intercourse increases each year. AIDS has become the fastest growing killer of both young men and young women. People living in larger cities are at greater risk than people in rural areas, but sexually active heterosexual men and women cannot consider themselves immune from HIV no matter where they live.

Is AIDS on the rise for heterosexual men and women?

There is a steady increase in the number of AIDS cases and HIV infections among heterosexual men and women in the United States. In 1989, more than 7,000 people with AIDS were infected with HIV from heterosexual sex. By 1995, the number had quadrupled, and in 2000 there were 78,000 people with AIDS who contracted HIV from heterosexual partners. Studies of HIV testing results have also shown an increasing number of infections among heterosexual men and women. The increase in heterosexual AIDS is because of

- the tendency for heterosexual people not to take precautions against HIV,
- resistance among heterosexual people against using condoms,
- the false beliefs that AIDS is a disease affecting only drug users and gay men, and
- the large number of HIV-infected, sexually active heterosexual people who do not know they are infected.

Are one-night stands risky for heterosexual people?

Yes. The less people know about their sex partner, the less aware they are about their risk for HIV. Research has shown that people are most likely to consider one-time sex partners risky and are more likely to use condoms with partners they do not know well. Because many heterosexual people who have HIV have not been tested, they are unaware of or are denying their risk. The more sex partners a person has, the greater the chances of having an HIV-positive partner.

Why are women at such high risk for HIV?

Women are at high risk for HIV infection for four main reasons:

- Women who inject drugs are at risk if they use needles and other injection equipment that was used by someone else. Injecting drugs accounts for more than 40% of all female AIDS patients in the United States.
- Women are at risk because of the men with whom they have sex. Forty percent of women with AIDS got HIV from a male sex partner.
- Women are at risk because the vagina is lined with mucous membranes, which are rich with blood vessels and cells that can be infected with HIV. Thus, women who have sexual intercourse with men who have been exposed to HIV are at high risk of HIV infection.
- Women often do not know the risk histories of their male sex partners.

What is the risk of getting HIV for survivors of rape and incest?

Survivors of rape and incest can be at high risk of HIV infection. However, the risk of HIV infection to sexual assault survivors depends entirely on the situation, and every situation is different. Sexual assault survivors are at greatest risk for HIV in large cities simply because there are more people with the virus in urban areas, making it more likely that the offender could be infected with HIV. Rape survivors, both men and women, are likely to be assaulted by men with a history of risky behaviors, including injecting drugs and having many sexual partners. Sex offenders are also likely to have prior criminal records. Spending time in prison, where injecting drugs and sex between inmates is common, can mean that a sex offender is infected with HIV at the time of his release from prison. Survivors should seek help in dealing with their assault, including getting tested for HIV and other sexually transmitted diseases (STDs).

Does infected semen stay in the vagina after intercourse to infect other men?

It is possible for HIV-infected semen to stay in the vagina after sex and pose a risk for infecting a subsequent sex partner. However, this is an unlikely route of HIV transmission.

Risky Partners and Risky Places

Risk of HIV infection comes from sexual partners and people who share injection drug equipment. Also, HIV is not equally prevalent in all places. The following questions pertain to situations that influence HIV transmission risks.

Who is "Patient Zero"?

Patient Zero is a generic term in the field of epidemiology that refers to the first case of a disease to which all others can be traced. In HIV, Patient Zero refers to a French-Canadian gay flight attendant who was among the first to be diagnosed with AIDS. In the early days of the HIV epidemic, health investigators from the Centers for Disease Control and Prevention identified sex partners who were either directly or indirectly infected through Patient Zero. Figure 4.1 shows the sexual contacts who were infected with HIV by Patient Zero. The reach of just a few sexual contacts within a short time illustrates the threat of HIV spreading among sex partners.

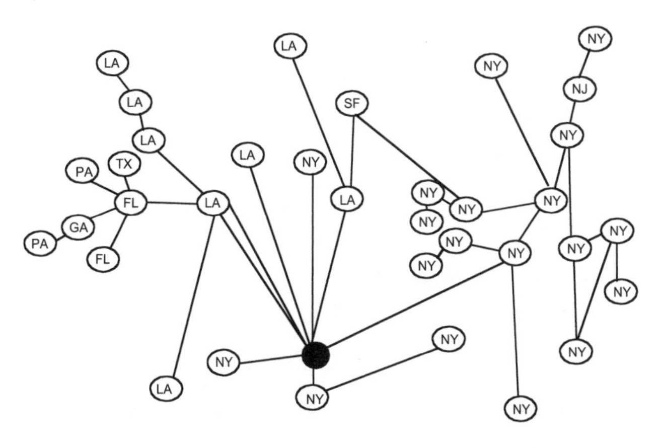

FIGURE 4.1. Sexual network of Patient Zero. The black circle represents Patient Zero, and each open circle represents an infected person. Letters in circles are state abbreviations.

What is a sex network?

Sex networks are the linkages between people who have sex with one another. The concept of a sexual network helps epidemiologists understand how an STD spreads in a population. Figure 4.1 provides an excellent example of a sexual network, in this case the sexual network of Patient Zero. Figure 4.2 depicts three sexual networks that have varying degrees of associated risks. Sex network A shows the risks for a monogamous person who is in a relationship with a partner who has three other partners, and two of those partners have other partners. In network B, a person may have a partner who is monogamous, but that person has another partner on the side who also has other partners. These two networks show the risk posed by relationships that are thought to be monogamous. Network C depicts a person who has five partners, most of whom also have multiple other partners.

Does the use of alcohol or other drugs increase the risk of HIV?

Yes. Drinking alcohol and using drugs can increase risk of HIV infection for the following reasons:

- People who are intoxicated are less likely to protect themselves from risks, including the risk of contracting HIV.
- Alcohol and other drugs change people's expectations about sex even when they are not intoxi-

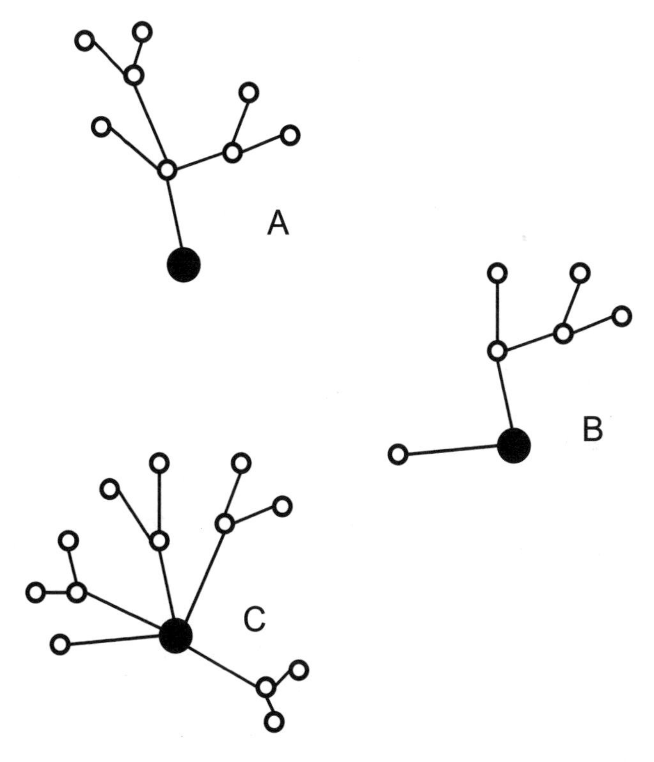

FIGURE 4.2. Sexual networks. A: Monogamous relationship for a person (represented by a black circle) whose partner has three other partners. B: Monogamous partner (represented by an open circle) whose partner has an extra-relationship partner who is not monogamous. C: Person who has five partners, most of whom also have multiple partners.

cated. People expect that they will take more risks and act more carelessly when they have been drinking.

- Alcohol and drugs can become a part of sexual relations, putting people at ease and increasing their willingness to do risky things.

However, drugs per se do not cause HIV infection unless the drugs or the equipment used to inject them are HIV contaminated. Instead, alcohol and drugs may promote risky behaviors in people who might not otherwise be at risk.

Can a person who got HIV from injecting drugs give the virus to sex partners?

It does not matter how the virus first gets into a person's body; it can be transmitted to others through different behaviors. People who get HIV from injecting drugs can pass the virus on to others through sex or continuing to share needles. Likewise, people who get HIV from having sex with infected partners can pass the virus on by sharing needles or continuing to have unsafe sex.

Can someone who has HIV infection but does not have symptoms of AIDS give the virus to others?

Yes. It takes most HIV-positive people years to develop symptoms. However, once infected with the virus, a person can transmit HIV to others. Although there is evidence that the virus is more rapidly transmitted in the early and later stages of HIV infection, HIV transmission can occur at any time in between, whether or not a person has symptoms.

How much risk is there for someone who has more than one sex partner?

People are put at risk not only by the number of sex partners they have. Having sexual intercourse with a single person who has HIV can cause HIV infection. However, having multiple sex partners means more opportunities to come in contact with one partner who has HIV. In studies of gay men, for example, those who had intercourse with five or more men had 18 times the risk of getting HIV compared with men who had a single male partner.

Is a person at risk if his or her spouse has had an affair?

Sexual encounters outside of long-term relationships run the risk of introducing STDs, including HIV, into the relationship. The virus is spread from one sex partner to another, so it is possible for someone to bring the virus home to his or her regular sex partner after getting it from an affair.

When is a couple considered monogamous?

Monogamy is defined as marriage with one person at a time, but it also applies to other types of relationships where two people are bonded. Monogamy can therefore mean that one person has one partner for life. On the other hand, monogamy can mean that a person has one partner at a time. In serial monogamy a person has several partners over time. A person who has serially monogamous relationships still has multiple sex partners, but they are not concurrent. When it comes to risk of HIV and other STDs, serial monogamy does not remove one's risk. Only when both partners know they do not have HIV and neither is injecting drugs or having sex with others does a monogamous relationship eliminate the risk of HIV infection.

Are people who live in certain parts of the United States at greater risk of HIV infection?

Yes. AIDS is not distributed evenly across the world or the United States. AIDS epidemics have spread at different rates in different places. The number of AIDS cases is greatest in the Northeastern and Southern United States, whereas AIDS cases have leveled off in some areas in the Midwest and West. People who live in New York City, Atlanta, or Miami and engage in high-risk drug use or sexual behavior are at greater risk of HIV than are people in Syracuse, NY, Macon, GA, or Pensacola, FL. However, the mere presence of HIV means that no one can be considered completely safe if he or she is engages in risky behaviors in places with lower rates of HIV.

Why are people who live in large cities at higher risk for HIV than people in small towns?

Throughout history, large cities have been hit hardest by epidemics, including the Black Plague that devastated 14th-century Europe and the cholera epidemic of the 1930s. Big cities are more likely to be densely populated, have poor health conditions, and have greater poverty, all of which help spread disease. In HIV epidemics, poverty is related to injecting drugs, which quickly spreads the virus. Relatively closed communities in cities have spread the virus in neighborhoods, areas, and districts, including gay and bisexual communities and the inner-city poor population. For these reasons, nearly 85% of all people with AIDS in the United States have lived in cities with populations greater than 500,000 people.

How many prostitutes have HIV infection?

It is impossible to know how many prostitutes (or any other groups of people) have been infected with HIV. Studies in some cities have found that many women and men who trade sex for money, drugs, or a place to stay are HIV positive. As one might expect, people involved in sex work in cities with the greatest number of people with AIDS also have the highest rate of HIV infection. In some areas of the world, such as some parts of Asia where drug use is prevalent and prostitution constitutes an important part of the social fabric, HIV is spreading rapidly.

How much risk is there from having sex with a female prostitute?

It is impossible to say that having sex with a prostitute will definitely result in HIV infection. Risk of infection depends on many factors, including the type of sex practiced, whether condoms are used, and geographical location. It is possible to have safe sex with a prostitute, so long as semen, vaginal fluids, or blood are not exchanged. Because prostitutes have many sex partners who themselves may have high-risk histories, prostitutes are considered to be at risk for HIV.

Do most prostitutes use condoms?

Research has shown that most prostitutes use condoms with their customers. However, it is also known that prostitutes are less likely to use condoms with their main sex partners. Thus, just like anyone else, if a prostitute has unprotected sex with a partner who has HIV, the prostitute is at high risk of getting the virus.

INFANTS, CHILDREN, ADOLESCENTS, AND ELDERLY PEOPLE

HIV infection is not a disease of any one particular type of person. The very young and the very old also become infected with HIV. However, the disease does seem to progress more rapidly in the underdeveloped immune system of infants and the frail immune system of elderly people.

Will a child born to an HIV-positive mother get AIDS?

Not every child born to a mother who has HIV becomes infected. The actual rates of HIV transmission during pregnancy vary, and the risk of infection during pregnancy and childbirth is reduced substantially when an HIV-positive mother undergoes HIV treatment. For this reason most women are advised to get tested for HIV if they plan to get pregnant or to get tested for HIV as a part of prenatal heath care.

How do children get AIDS?

The majority of children with AIDS get infected with HIV by their mother during pregnancy, delivery, or breast-feeding. As of the year 2000, there had been more than 8,800 children in the United States with AIDS, and more than 90% of those children got the virus from their HIV-positive mother.

Why are adolescents at high risk for HIV?

More than 25,000 males and 12,000 females younger than age 25 have been diagnosed with AIDS in the United States. An additional 89,000 people between the ages of 25 and 29 have been diagnosed with AIDS. Because it takes an average of 8 to 10 years for HIV infection to develop into AIDS, the majority of these people became infected in their teens. More than half of high school students have sexual intercourse in short-term relationships. Therefore, when HIV is introduced into an adolescent peer group, it can rapidly spread. Teenage pregnancies and the number of other STDs among adolescents testify to the likelihood that adolescents are at risk of getting HIV infection.

Are elderly people at risk for HIV?

Senior citizens were frequent recipients of blood transfusions before the blood supply was deemed safe. At that time, the elderly population was at risk of HIV infection and proceeded to transmit the virus to their sex partners. Because the blood supply is now safe, elderly people are no longer at risk of HIV infection from blood transfusions. However, the growing population of older people living with HIV creates greater risk for older people who form new sexual relationships. As of the year 2000, 6% of men and 5% of women with AIDS were ages 55 or older at the time of diagnosis. As people with HIV infection continue to live longer and healthier lives because of effective treatments, the population of older people with HIV will continue to grow.

SUMMARY

Risk for HIV is not as much a matter of who a person is as what a person does. It was once easy to think about groups of people being at risk of HIV infection. Today, anyone who engages in behaviors that could cause exposure to the virus is at risk. People at greatest risk include

- anyone who has shared needles or other equipment to inject drugs,
- any person who has ever had sex with someone who injects drugs,
- men who have had anal intercourse with another man,
- women who have had sex with a man who has had sex with other men,
- people who have had other STDs,
- men and women who have had sex with a prostitute, and
- any person who has a sex partner who engages in or has engaged in unprotected sex.

Although most situations that create risk for HIV are now well understood, people try to minimize their concern about the highest risk behaviors and overestimate the risk of situations that are virtually free of risk. For example, the risk of dying in a plane crash can appear greater than that of a car accident, when actually the opposite is true. People have many questions about situations that create little risk for HIV infection, and these questions are the focus of chapter 5.

5

Can I Get AIDS From . . . ?

The vast majority of people with AIDS were HIV infected from having sex or sharing needles with an HIV-positive partner. Babies born to HIV-infected mothers and people who received untested blood transfusions also account for many AIDS cases. And then there are some unusual ways in which one or maybe two people may have been infected with HIV. Freak accidents attract our attention because they are novel and overshadow the familiar day-to-day realities of AIDS. Contracting HIV is theoretically possible when a person comes in contact with the virus. These situations illustrate theoretical risks, situations in which it is possible to get HIV, although the actual risk is small. Many questions arise about situations with theoretical risk, and many related questions stem from AIDS myths. Exhibit 5.1 summarizes some common HIV transmission myths identified in the United States. This chapter answers questions about circumstances that have caused concern about getting HIV but in reality have little or no risk for HIV transmission.

EXHIBIT 5.1. HIV Transmission Myths and Facts

Myth	*Fact*
HIV is not the cause of AIDS.	HIV destroys the immune system and causes AIDS.
All people who have HIV look sick.	Most people with HIV look and feel healthy.
You can get AIDS by kissing someone with HIV.	HIV is spread by anal, vaginal, and oral sex.
Only sexually promiscuous people get AIDS.	Anyone who practices unsafe behaviors can get HIV.
If my sex partner loves me, he or she will be true to me.	Even loving partners can have sex outside of relationships.
Condoms do not protect people from HIV.	Latex condoms are effective in preventing HIV and other sexually transmitted diseases.
An HIV-positive person who has an undetectable viral load cannot infect others.	An undetectable viral load means that the virus has slowed its growth but is not eliminated.
There is a cure for AIDS.	There is not yet a cure for AIDS.

Blood Transfusions and Organ Transplants

A blood transfusion with HIV-infected blood is the most dangerous situation for HIV infection. Virtually every person who had an HIV-contaminated blood transfusion became HIV infected. Fortunately, effective blood-screening techniques have removed the risk of getting HIV from blood transfusions.

How safe is it to get a blood transfusion?

Blood transfusions are now very safe. The risk of receiving HIV-infected blood during a blood transfusion in the United States is extremely low because people with high-risk histories are dissuaded from donating blood, and all donated blood is tested for HIV antibodies. The only way that infected blood could get into the blood supply is if an HIV-infected person donated blood during the window period before he or she developed antibodies against HIV. It is estimated that HIV-infected blood may escape detection in less than 1 in 60,000 donations, accounting for only a small fraction of the millions of blood donations received each year. Risks vary in different places; greater risks occur in large metropolitan areas where there are more people with HIV infection. HIV screening programs are expensive, so some developing countries where HIV is prevalent still do not have universal screening for HIV, making blood transfusions in developing countries more risky than in developed countries.

When did it become safe to have a blood transfusion?

In the early 1980s, medical professionals first realized that people were becoming infected with what was at the time an unknown virus through blood transfusions. In 1983, attempts were made to screen blood donors for possible risk histories through donor deferral programs. Donor screening was somewhat successful in improving the safety of the blood supply but could not remove infected blood once it slipped through. In 1985, the first test for detecting HIV antibodies became available and was immediately used to screen donated blood. The greatest risk for HIV infection through blood transfusions in the United States therefore occurred between the late 1970s, when the HIV epidemic first started in the United States, and 1985, when universal blood screening was established.

Can people receive their own blood during an operation to avoid getting HIV and other blood diseases?

Yes, they can store their own blood ahead of time and use it for surgery. Using one's own blood is an option that is particularly important for people with rare blood types or other factors that limit their ability to receive donated blood. Another option is for a person to receive blood donated from a friend or relative who has the same blood type. However, today blood banks are safe, and it is not necessary to donate one's own blood to avoid HIV.

Why did so many individuals with hemophilia get AIDS?

Hemophilia is an inherited disease that causes uncontrolled bleeding. Blood diseases like hemophilia are treated by replacing missing clotting factors with clotting factors obtained from multiple donors. People with blood-clotting diseases became infected with HIV before high-risk donors were identified and donated blood was screened for HIV antibodies. In the early 1980s, before a test for HIV was available, more than half of all individuals with hemophilia in the United States became HIV infected. Indeed, AIDS had become a more lethal threat to them than the clotting disease itself. Fortunately, testing for HIV antibodies has made blood transfusions safe and has removed most of these risks.

Can a person get AIDS from having an organ or tissue transplant?

Organs and tissues donated from a person with HIV infection contain the virus and can infect recipients. For this reason, the same procedures used for screening donated blood are used for tissue and organ donations. The odds are small that a person would get HIV from organ and body tissue transplants in the United States. However, other countries have not been as diligent as the United States about screening and testing for HIV. Biomedical products that contain human tissue produced outside of the United States should be carefully traced and tested to avoid possible infection.

Is it possible to get HIV from donating (giving) blood?

No. The association between blood donation and HIV infection is a one-way street. People can only be infected with HIV by getting blood, not from giving blood. It is impossible for a person to get HIV from donating blood in the United States because all of the equipment is sealed sterile for each donor and disposed of after each donation. Needles can cause infection only when they are contaminated with HIV, and this is not possible when a sterile needle is used for each donor.

Are blood donors informed of the HIV screening test results?

All donated blood in the United States is tested for HIV antibodies. People who donate blood that tests negative for HIV antibodies are not informed that they are not infected. In this case, no news is good news. Blood that tests HIV positive, or positive for several blood diseases, is traced back to donors, who are contacted and referred for further testing and services.

HEALTH CARE WORKERS

Working in hospitals and clinics can expose health care professionals to blood and other potentially infectious body fluids. However, medical and dental professionals can and should protect themselves from exposure to disease. Wearing latex gloves, sterilizing instruments, and disinfecting medical equipment helps protect professionals as well as their patients. In rare situations, however, occupational accidents occur in which medical providers are infected with HIV (see

TABLE 5.1. HIV Infections Among Health Care Workers Caused by Occupational Exposure

Health occupation	*Cases known*	*Cases presumed*
Dentist–dental workers	0	6
Emergency medical technician	0	12
Health aide	1	15
Housekeeper–maintenance	2	12
Lab technician	19	17
Nurse	23	35
Physician	6	18
Respiratory therapist	1	2
Patient care technician	4	7

the cases in Table 5.1). The most cases of health professionals infected with HIV through occupational exposures have occurred among nurses and physicians.

Can professionals who draw blood from individuals with HIV get the virus if they get stuck with a needle?

Needle-stick injuries are the most common type of health care occupational accident. Professional blood drawers (phlebotomists) experience a needle-stick injury about once in every 600 times they draw blood. Needle sticks usually happen when putting the protective cap back on a used needle. For HIV infection to occur, the phlebotomist must get stuck with a needle after drawing blood from a person infected with the virus. But even then the chances of HIV infection are between 1 in 200 and 1 in 1,000! One study of 1,534 health care workers who were exposed to HIV-infected blood, most by needle sticks, found that only two people became infected. Nevertheless, phlebotomists and other professionals who draw blood should wear latex gloves to provide an extra layer of protection.

Should a professional who draws blood wear gloves?

Yes. All health care professionals who draw blood or come in contact with blood are advised to wear latex gloves for their own protection as well as to protect their patients. This is true not only for protection against HIV but also to control the spread of many diseases. Latex gloves cover small cuts and abrasions in the skin, wipe exterior blood off a needle as it passes through the latex, and provide a sterile barrier between the provider and patient.

Should people worry about whether their dentist has HIV infection?

People are particularly wary of being treated by an HIV-positive dentist. News coverage in the 1980s of six people who got infected from one Florida dentist caused alarm about the potential danger of HIV infection in dental practices. Genetic testing showed that the infections were caused by a strain of HIV carried by that particular dentist himself—the instruments were contaminated by the dentist's own blood, not the blood of his patients. It is still not known whether the dentist deliberately or accidentally infected these patients. However, these six people are the only recorded cases of HIV infection caused by an HIV-infected dentist. Still, the American Dental Association established guidelines for dental practice after the Florida incident. In general, dentists who are HIV positive are not supposed to practice invasive procedures that could carry the risk that their patients will come into contact with their blood.

Can a person get AIDS from the instruments and tools that a dentist uses?

Because dental instruments come in direct contact with blood, HIV-contaminated dental instruments could cause infection. However, HIV is easily destroyed when instruments are sterilized. Dentists routinely sterilize their instruments between patients, and there is no risk of HIV transmission from sterilized instruments.

Can a person get HIV from kidney dialysis or other medical procedures?

Any situation that can expose a person's bloodstream to the virus can cause HIV infection. Kidney dialysis filters blood when the kidneys themselves are unable to do so. If dialysis equipment is not cleaned between patients, it is possible that a person could become HIV infected from a patient who was previously treated. However, HIV infections caused by contaminated medical equipment and instruments in developed countries are extremely rare. On the other hand, in developing countries with poorly resourced medical care, disease transmission including HIV infection in medical settings does occur. For example, nuclear medicine procedures that involve injecting materials into the bloodstream have resulted in a few cases of HIV infection in the world out of more than 38 million such procedures conducted each year.

Can a nurse's aide get HIV from coming in contact with body fluids of people with HIV or AIDS?

All health care professionals should be cautious in situations in which they could be exposed to a patient's blood. However, HIV-infected blood can enter the body only through an opening in the skin or through contact with mucous membranes. As of 1999, there were only 56 health professionals in the United States who were known to be infected with HIV while on the job and another 124 who may have been HIV infected. Professionals who appear to be at greatest risk include nurses, laboratory technicians who handle blood samples, and doctors. In almost every case where a professional has been infected, infection occurred because of a cut caused by an HIV-contaminated instrument. Although just one case of HIV infection is too many, the fact that so few health care professionals have been infected, out of the millions who provide daily care to people with HIV, shows how rare these cases are.

Can doctors or dentists require that their patients be tested for HIV before treating them?

No. HIV testing requires a patient's informed consent and like any other medical examination or test, doctors cannot force patients to get tested. Doctors who advise patients to get tested do so as they would for any other medical test. A doctor cannot ethically refuse to treat people who are HIV positive, and they cannot refuse to treat people who do not want to get tested.

Do doctors or dentists have to tell their patients that they are HIV positive?

No. Doctors do not have to disclose their health status to their patients, and that includes their HIV status. However, doctors with HIV are responsible for not doing procedures that could place their patients at risk. The American Medical Association has specifically stated that any physician who knows that he or she has an infectious disease should not engage in any activity that creates risk of transmission of the disease to others.

Occupational Hazards

For many people, their job involves close contact with coworkers. Often when one person at work gets sick, the bug spreads throughout the workplace. Fear of a devastating disease like HIV infection can cause people who work with an HIV-positive person to feel unsafe.

If a coworker has AIDS, can a person get HIV from sharing work materials, equipment, the phone, or other objects on the job?

HIV does not exist on surfaces or objects. It is impossible to get HIV from sharing equipment or materials with an HIV-infected coworker. HIV cannot be spread by sharing a phone with a person who has the virus or by working in a confined physical space with an HIV-positive person.

Can people give HIV to their hairdressers?

People often get nicked or cut during a haircut. If a person with HIV bleeds during a haircut, direct contact with blood must be avoided. Unless there is direct contact with blood, however, there is no risk of contracting HIV. Likewise, a person can only get HIV from a hairdresser who is HIV positive if that hairdresser gets cut and bleeds on the customer, particularly if blood gets on a mucous membrane.

Can a person get HIV if a coworker gets cut or injured?

Direct contact with human blood always carries some risk of HIV infection as well as other diseases. For HIV infection to occur, an ample amount of blood must enter a person's body. Thus, it is possible that direct contact with blood while on the job can cause HIV infection, but it would be extremely unusual. For example, if an HIV-positive person were injured and bled on a coworker who had an open cut or sore that came in contact with infected blood, it is possible, although still unlikely, that the coworker could get HIV.

Is it possible for a person to get HIV from cleaning blood-stained carpeting or clothes?

Cleaning blood, either fresh or dry, should always be done with caution. However, HIV does not remain viable for long, and detergents destroy the virus. Wearing gloves and using cleaning solutions removes the risks of HIV infection from cleaning dried blood.

Human Bites

A human bite that pierces the skin and causes bleeding can be a dangerous source of infection because of the many bacteria and viruses that exist in saliva. Because HIV has been found in saliva, questions arise as to whether a person can get HIV through a bite. Human bites occur in only a few situations, such as unusually aggressive fights, attacks from someone with mental illness, attacks on police and emergency workers, or bites from small children.

Can a person get the virus if he or she is bitten by someone who has HIV or AIDS?

HIV itself and HIV-infected immune cells can exist in saliva. It is theoretically possible that exposing the bloodstream to saliva could cause HIV infection. However, it is unlikely that infectable cells would be exposed to a sufficient amount of HIV during a human bite. One study followed 13 people bitten by someone with HIV, and none of them became infected. In another study of 30 emergency room doctors and nurses who were bitten or scratched by aggressive HIV-positive patients, not one got HIV. In fact, there have been very few documented cases of people infected with HIV through human bites.

Can a person get HIV if he or she bites someone who has the virus?

Exposing the mucous membranes to HIV-infected blood carries the risk of getting HIV infection. Even a small amount of HIV infected blood can be sufficient for infection. Although infection from biting a person with HIV is possible, it is also very unlikely.

Is it possible for children to get HIV if they are bitten by a child who has HIV?

Much of the concern about human bites involves children, usually small children who are teething. Biting is a common problem with small children and causes concern regardless of whether a child has HIV infection. It is not likely that a child could transmit HIV to another child unless there was exposure to blood.

Schools

Parents generally wish to protect their children. Knowing that a school has an HIV-positive student can cause some parents to be alarmed about the safety of their children, especially when parents are misinformed about how HIV is transmitted. One survey showed that less than half of parents are willing to allow their children to stay in the same schoolroom with a child who is HIV-positive. Discrimination against children with HIV has been one of the darkest sides of the AIDS epidemic. The story of Ryan White, a young boy who had HIV and was discriminated against by his school, showed how hurtful the irrational fear of AIDS can be to children.

Ryan White was 14 years old when he was diagnosed with AIDS as a result of treatment for hemophilia with blood-clotting agents. He was removed from school because of irrational fears, and he suffered ridicule about having AIDS. Ultimately, he won the right to return to school through a series of legal battles and became an international icon for AIDS education.

Are small children who attend school with an HIV-positive child at risk of getting the virus?

HIV cannot be transmitted from child to child through sharing toys, school supplies, playground or bathroom facilities, or close physical contact. Even sharing food or teething toys does not pose risk for transmitting HIV. Although preschoolers do have lots of contact that often involves saliva, there are no known cases of child-to-child HIV transmission. The only way that a child could be at risk for HIV in school is through direct contact with the blood of an HIV-positive child.

What could put children at risk of getting HIV if their schoolmates have the virus?

In a few rare situations, a child with HIV could transmit the virus to other children. Injuries, such as accidents, cuts, or fights that produce bleeding, could expose other children to the virus. But it is necessary for a child to have direct contact with infected blood, a situation that should be avoided whether or not a child has HIV.

Do foster parents who care for children with HIV have to do anything to protect themselves or their family from getting the virus?

Children born with HIV infection often lose their mothers to AIDS and are orphaned at a young age. Thus, it is not uncommon for children with HIV to require foster care. Having a child with HIV in the home does not place a foster family at risk. Special attention is required only if a child bleeds. Latex gloves, detergents, and disinfectants remove the risks of infection when there is blood to be dealt with from cuts, scrapes, and other injuries.

Sharp Objects

Any object that has come in contact with HIV-infected blood that subsequently comes in contact with another person's mucous membranes or bloodstream can cause HIV infection. Thus, sharp objects that pierce the skin can create the risk of transmitting the virus.

Is it possible to get HIV from wearing a pair of earrings that belongs to someone with HIV?

Cleaning detergents can be used to disinfect earrings and destroy HIV. In addition, HIV infection can only result when a person is exposed to a sufficient amount of blood that contains a minimum dose of the virus. Thus, it is not possible for HIV transmission to occur by sharing earrings, assuming there is no blood on their surface. HIV is a fragile virus, so simply cleaning earrings with a disinfectant removes all risks of HIV transmission.

Is there any risk of HIV infection from getting a tattoo?

Tattoos use hollow needles to infuse ink under the skin. If needles are reused, it is possible to transmit HIV. But the risk of HIV infection is small because blood is not drawn into tattooing needles and ink is placed just under the skin. However, because dirty needles can cause other infections, needles must be discarded after a single use.

Can a person get HIV by stepping on a hypodermic needle?

Dirty injection needles can carry enough HIV to cause infection. Because used needles can also transmit infections other than HIV, including tetanus and hepatitis, a doctor should examine injuries caused by dirty needles. Needles found in public places such as parks and beaches should be handled with particular caution. Local health departments should be called to safely dispose of hazardous materials like dirty needles.

Is there any risk of getting HIV if a person shares a razor with someone who has the virus?

Razors can nick skin and cause bleeding. Although it is possible that HIV could be transmitted if blood remains on a razor that is used by a second person who also gets cut, it is unlikely that a sufficient amount of blood could be present to cause infection. Therefore, the risk is extremely small for contracting HIV from an HIV-positive person's razor.

Can a person get the virus if he or she uses a knife that someone else got cut on?

For a knife to transmit HIV from one person to another, infected blood would have to enter the bloodstream of another person. This would be an unusual accident. Once a knife has been cleaned, it is not possible for HIV to be passed on this way.

Bloody Contacts

Direct contact with HIV-contaminated blood is the riskiest situation for transmission of HIV infection. However, blood that comes in contact with intact skin does not cause infection. Small openings in the skin such as cuts, scrapes, and lesions can allow HIV to enter the bloodstream and cause infection, so any contact with the blood of an HIV-positive person is potentially risky.

Is it risky to clean glass that a person with HIV got cut on?

Cleaning bloody glass is very risky if the blood has HIV. Great care should be taken in situations such as these so as not to get cut while handling HIV-positive blood or other materials. Wearing latex or rubber gloves and using proper detergents offers the best protection against HIV infection.

Can a person be at risk for HIV if someone's blood gets on his or her skin?

The skin has a protective outer layer of cells that keeps HIV and other viruses from gaining access to immune cells. Contact between blood and intact skin carries no risk of HIV transmission. However, it is possible for HIV to enter a cut, sore, or other wound that comes in direct contact with HIV-infected blood.

Is there risk of HIV infection from contact sports, like football, basketball, or boxing?

In many sports, athletes may have injuries that bleed. High-contact sports can allow exposure to blood that, if infected with HIV, could transmit infection to another player. However, HIV must have access to mucous membranes or the bloodstream. One study showed that risk of HIV infection among professional football players is less than 1 in 85 million game contacts. In contrast, however, boxing often involves significant amounts of blood and multiple cuts that could allow access to the bloodstream. Trainers, coaches, and medics who care for athletic injuries may have direct contact with blood and should always practice good infection control, including wearing latex gloves. In the absence of blood, contact sports have no risk of HIV transmission.

If someone gets in an accident and is bleeding, is it possible to get AIDS from helping them?

There is a risk of getting HIV whenever a person comes in direct contact with blood. Helping an accident victim is no exception. However, it is possible to help accident victims without concern for getting HIV if there is no direct contact with blood. Even mouth-to-mouth resuscitation does not carry the risk of HIV infection unless the person is bleeding.

Can a person get AIDS from handling a dirty bandage?

Dirty bandages should always be handled with caution. However, it is unlikely that HIV infection could occur from handling a contaminated bandage, unless it was saturated with infected blood and the blood came in direct contact with an opening in the skin.

Sharing Facilities

Some viruses and bacteria are spread from person-to-object-to-person. Fortunately, it is impossible to transmit HIV by way of objects unless blood is present. Knowing that some diseases can spread through indirect contact, however, raises questions about HIV.

Is it possible to get HIV from a public restroom, by using a toilet after someone with HIV has used it, or from touching surfaces like a doorknob after someone with AIDS?

No. HIV infection occurs only when a sufficient amount of the virus enters the body. Because small amounts of HIV have been found in urine and feces, contamination of toilet seats is unlikely. Even if a person sits in blood on a toilet seat—a worst-case scenario—there would have to be an open cut on the skin to allow HIV access to the bloodstream. Thus, HIV transmission cannot occur from using a restroom previously used by someone with HIV infection. The same is true for doorknobs and other surfaces.

Can a person get HIV from a public swimming pool or hot tub?

No. HIV is a delicate virus. Chlorinated water in swimming pools and hot tubs destroys HIV.

If a person gets cut while working out at a health club, can HIV be contracted if the equipment was previously used by a person with AIDS?

No. HIV does not mysteriously drift from objects into a person's body. A cut does not just pick up HIV. It is not possible for a person to get HIV through a cut that touches a surface touched by a person with AIDS.

Is it possible to get HIV from sharing laundry facilities?

HIV cannot be contracted by handling clothes worn by an HIV-infected person. The virus cannot remain in washing machines or dryers and cannot be passed on to clothes that are later washed or dried.

Sharing Spaces

Living with someone who has HIV infection can cause concern about getting the virus. As people with AIDS get sicker, they rely on others for their care. For this reason, researchers have studied the risk of getting HIV from living with someone who has the virus. Results from these studies answer questions about the risks from living with a person who has HIV.

Can a person get HIV from sharing a home with a person who has AIDS?

No. Studies conducted with people who live with someone who has AIDS have examined risks related to close living arrangements. People who provide hands-on care and are exposed to body fluids on a daily basis have also been carefully observed. Caretakers share eating utensils, bathroom facilities, and all other aspects of home life. These studies have consistently shown that people who do not engage in sexual acts with infected housemates and do not come in direct contact with their blood do not become HIV infected.

Can a person get HIV from cleaning house for a person who has AIDS?

Contact with the body fluids of someone with HIV cannot cause infection unless there is a significant amount of exposure through a skin opening. All of the precautions that should be taken when cleaning dried blood, such as wearing latex gloves and avoiding direct contact, offer protection against infection. Situations like housecleaning that do not involve contact with blood pose no risk of HIV infection.

Can a person get HIV from sharing a toothbrush with someone who has AIDS?

Sharing toothbrushes can spread germs. However, there is so little HIV found in saliva, and HIV is so sensitive to detergents, such as those found in toothpaste, that it is not possible for a person to get HIV from sharing a toothbrush. Still, it is probably wise not to share toothbrushes, because many other diseases can be passed on this way.

Is there risk from sharing makeup with a person who has HIV?

Sharing makeup can spread disease, particularly viruses and bacteria that infect the eyes. Conjunctivitis is just one example of a contagious eye disease. But it is not possible for HIV to be spread by sharing makeup.

Are children in the family of a person living with AIDS at risk of getting the virus?

A common reaction in families with a person who has HIV infection is to keep them away from children. Isolating HIV-positive people from children is one of the most hurtful experiences for people with HIV. There is no risk for children getting HIV through casual contact with HIV-positive people.

Touching

The most obvious way to distance people with AIDS is to deprive them of human touch. Physical contact provides a sense of closeness. Touch can be a form of support and human connection, and touching a person with HIV carries no risk of HIV transmission.

Can a person get HIV from touching someone who has AIDS?

No. It is impossible to get HIV from merely touching someone infected with the virus. HIV does not penetrate skin and must have access to infectable cells for infection to occur. Even close contact that goes on for a long time, such as hand holding, hugging, or embracing, does not pose any risk of HIV transmission.

Can HIV be transmitted through tears?

HIV has been found in small amounts in human tears. However, it is not possible to transmit HIV through contact with tears because not enough active virus particles are present. In addition, proteins found in tears are known to kill the virus. Wiping away the tears of someone who has AIDS does not present a risk of contracting the virus.

Does a massage therapist have to worry about getting HIV from clients who have AIDS?

People with AIDS often seek massage therapy as a part of healing and coping. Touching the skin of someone with AIDS cannot cause HIV infection as long as there is no direct contact with open sores or wounds.

Is there any risk of getting HIV if someone touches a lesion caused by a skin infection or Kaposi's sarcoma?

Direct contact with open wounds should always be avoided whether or not the person has HIV. When a caretaker helps someone with HIV or AIDS treat an open sore, such as those that can occur with Kaposi's sarcoma, latex gloves should always be worn and disinfectants should be used to protect against HIV transmission.

Near-Sex Experiences

Vaginal and anal intercourse are the most common sources of HIV infection. However, sex involves much more than penetrating acts. Sexual contact that does not involve intercourse can still include very close contact with body fluids and can raise the specter of HIV infection.

Can people get HIV if their sex partners ejaculate on their skin but not in their body?

Semen can contain high concentrations of HIV and HIV-infected immune cells. However, the skin provides a protective barrier against the virus. It is therefore not possible to get HIV from direct contact with semen placed on the body but not in the body.

Can people get HIV from an exotic dancer who comes really close to them or rubs up against them?

Close does not count when it comes to HIV transmission. Assuming that the dancer does in fact have HIV infection, just being near a person is not enough to get the virus.

Is it possible to get HIV from nibbling on a sex partner's ear lobe?

People can have intimate contact with each other without any risk of getting or giving HIV. It is impossible to get the virus from sexual contact that does not involve the exchange of semen, vaginal fluids, or blood in such a way that a sufficient amount of the virus gets into the body. Nibbling, kissing, or caressing cannot cause HIV infection.

Eating, Drinking, and Smoking

Sharing utensils, cups, and glasses can mean getting someone's saliva on the lips and mouth. Taken literally, this would mean mucous membrane contact with saliva that could contain HIV. For many people, the prospect of getting or giving HIV through eating and drinking causes unnecessary alarm.

Does sharing a drinking cup, glass, or food with someone who has HIV spread the virus?

No. Sharing drinks and food can pass on other germs from person to person, but HIV cannot be spread this way. It is not possible for a sufficient amount of HIV to gain access to the body of a person who shares a drinking glass or cup or eating utensils with someone who has the virus.

Is it possible for a cook who has AIDS to pass on the virus through food?

Food prepared by someone with HIV cannot transmit the virus. HIV could not even be transmitted in a freak accident in which a person with HIV was cut while preparing food unless there were quite a bit of blood. However, other diseases such as hepatitis A can be transmitted through food.

Can sharing cigarettes with a person who has AIDS spread HIV?

Sharing cigarettes cannot spread HIV because there is not enough virus present in saliva to cause infection. Smoking tobacco causes many deadly diseases, but HIV infection is not one of them.

Insects and Animals

The connection between HIV and animals is confusing. There has been much discussion about whether

HIV is carried from person to insect to person and whether animals can get and give HIV infection.

Can mosquitoes carry HIV from person to person?

No. Mosquitoes can carry other diseases that cause sickness and death in humans, such as malaria, meningitis, and West Nile Virus infection. In these cases, the mosquito is part of the life cycle of the disease and acts as a natural carrier. It was once feared that insects that first bite an HIV-infected person could then transmit the virus to others. The idea originated from the high rates of AIDS found in central Florida, where mosquitos are abundant. Despite these early scares, studies have shown that HIV does not complete its viral cycle in insect cells, making mosquitoes an impossible carrier for HIV. Furthermore, the amount of blood residue on a mosquito stinger is not sufficient for HIV transmission because insects ingest blood, they do not inject it. Studies in areas with both high rates of AIDS and dense mosquito populations, like central Florida, have shown that HIV infection is unrelated to mosquito bites; elderly people and children do not have high rates of HIV infection even when they suffer multiple mosquito bites.

If someone who has AIDS has a pet dog or cat that has fleas, is it possible for the fleas to carry the virus and transmit it?

No. Fleas, like mosquitoes, cannot harbor HIV and cannot pass the virus to people.

Do cats carry the virus that causes AIDS?

No. There is a virus that causes severe immune suppression in cats called *feline immunodeficiency virus* (FIV). This virus ultimately causes cats to get a disease like AIDS. FIV is a retrovirus like HIV, and both FIV and HIV cause diseases in similar ways. However, FIV cannot cause AIDS in humans, and HIV cannot cause disease in cats.

If a dog or cat bites someone with HIV, can the virus be passed on to another person?

HIV only exists in human cells. It is therefore not possible for a dog or cat to be a carrier for HIV.

What animals can carry HIV and pass it on to humans?

There are viruses like HIV that cause infections leading to diseases like AIDS in other animals. Visna virus found in sheep, FIV in cats, simian immunodeficiency virus in apes, and avian sarcoma virus in chickens are some examples. However, none of these viruses causes disease in humans, and animals do not carry HIV.

Summary

Many of the questions in this chapter stem from AIDS myths, culturally held beliefs about AIDS that are not grounded in fact. Fears of getting HIV from common, daily experiences such as work accidents, public phones, donating blood, or going to a dentist become exaggerated to the point where rare events that have no real risk appear more threatening than common high-risk situations. Similarly, airline crashes can seem threatening and cause fear, whereas the chances of dying in an auto accident are far greater than dying in a plane crash. It is a psychological fact that vivid emotional images, such as those that follow an air accident, can make remote risks seem more threatening. There is virtually no risk that a child with HIV could infect another child, but rumors fuel irrational fears and panic, which in turn lead to prejudice. One of the great ironies of the AIDS epidemic is that people worry about getting HIV from their dentist but shrug off risks that arise from having unprotected sexual intercourse. Focusing attention on improbable risks allows people to avoid dealing with more likely and immediate threats.

6

What Should I Know About HIV Testing?

People can find out whether they are infected with HIV only by taking an HIV test. When AIDS was first identified in 1981, doctors did not know what was causing the immune system damage that resulted in AIDS. By 1983, HIV itself was discovered. Researchers were then able to grow the virus in laboratories, a critical step in understanding the workings of the virus. These discoveries paved the way for the first test for HIV, developed in 1985. Today, HIV testing is one of the cornerstones of international efforts to stop AIDS. Approximately 24.6 million people in the United States are tested for HIV each year. Yet people have many questions about the HIV test. In fact, of all of the questions asked of AIDS hotline workers, the most common questions concern HIV testing.

The HIV Test

HIV testing determines whether a person has been infected with the virus that causes AIDS. Although most people know that testing is available, they often have questions about the testing procedure.

What is the AIDS test?

AIDS is the end-stage of HIV infection. A person with AIDS has a severely depleted immune system and usually has been diagnosed with at least one of several life-threatening illnesses. AIDS is therefore a medical diagnosis based on symptoms of infections, cancers, or immune suppression. Many blood tests are used to guide the treatment of people with AIDS, including T-helper lymphocyte cell counts and viral load tests. However, a person who is diagnosed with AIDS must also have HIV infection, which is determined only by HIV testing.

What is the HIV test?

HIV testing determines whether a person has been infected with HIV. Some tests for HIV infection involve detecting the virus directly in the bloodstream. However, tests that determine the presence of HIV itself are relatively expensive and require special laboratories equipped to directly handle the virus. The most widely used tests for HIV infection detect antibodies to HIV rather than the presence of the virus itself. Antibodies are produced by the immune system in response to an invading virus or other causes of disease. Each foreign particle that the immune system attacks is assigned its own specific antibody. Antibodies for one virus cannot be easily confused with antibodies produced for a different virus. Therefore, the presence of specific antibodies means that a person has been exposed to a specific virus.

Can a person be exposed to HIV and not test HIV positive?

Yes. People can be exposed to HIV and not become infected. For example, a person may have unprotected sex with an HIV-positive partner—therefore being exposed to HIV—and not become infected. Only when a person becomes infected with HIV and produces antibodies against HIV will the person test HIV positive.

How many tests are done during HIV testing?

HIV testing involves the following steps:

- A person interested in getting tested is told about the test, what it consists of, and what the results mean (pretest counseling).
- The person must consent to the test voluntarily.
- Vials of blood are drawn just as they would be for any other type of blood test.
- The blood is sent to a laboratory that does the actual HIV testing.
- The first test done is a sensitive screening test for HIV antibodies. If this test does not detect the presence of HIV antibodies, the test is complete

and the person is considered to be HIV negative; antibodies for HIV are not present. If the screening test is positive, antibodies for HIV may be present, and the screening test is repeated once again.

- If the second screening test is positive, a second type of test is done to confirm that the screening tests really did detect HIV antibodies.

Thus, one test is done when no HIV antibodies are detected, but two types of tests are conducted when the screening test does detect antibodies.

What is the ELISA test?

Blood drawn for HIV testing is first screened for HIV antibodies using an enzyme-linked immunosorbent assay (ELISA) test. ELISA is one of several techniques available for antibody testing. The ELISA test is done first because it is sensitive to HIV antibodies—if HIV antibodies are present, the ELISA test is likely to detect them. A negative ELISA test (i.e., when the test does not detect HIV antibodies) is very unlikely to be wrong. However, positive ELISA tests are always repeated because the test can mistakenly pick up non-HIV antibodies. For this reason, the ELISA test is used to first screen blood for the presence of HIV antibodies.

What is the Western blot test?

Western blot tests are also used for detecting HIV antibodies; it is the confirmatory test that is performed when the ELISA test is positive. A Western blot test will determine the exact antigens, or parts of HIV, that HIV antibodies target. A positive Western blot result, where HIV antibodies have been detected, means that two out of three precise antigens from components of HIV have been identified. Western blot specifically tests for the presence of antibodies against three groups of proteins that are part of HIV: the proteins that form the viral envelope, a group of proteins found in the core of the virus, and the polymerase enzyme that is essential for the replication of HIV. At least two of the three antibodies must be present in a person's blood for a positive Western blot test. Detection of antibodies against certain viral proteins makes the Western blot test specific to HIV and confirms the results of an ELISA test. For a diagnosis of HIV infection, it is necessary to have both positive ELISA and Western blot tests.

How are ELISA and Western blot tests similar and different?

Both the ELISA and Western blot are used to detect antibodies to viruses and other causes of disease. They are serological tests, meaning they are both used to analyze the fluid portion of blood called *serum*. (Blood serum is the same as blood plasma but without the proteins that cause blood clotting.) The ELISA procedure detects antibodies that the body produces to fight the virus. Western blot tests, however, determine the specific antigen, or part of the virus, to which the antibody is targeted. The Western blot test is therefore more precise because it identifies specific antigens. Another difference between ELISA and Western blot tests is cost; Western blot tests are more expensive than ELISA tests. Western blot also takes a longer time for results. ELISA testing is better suited for automated processing that allows labs to run more tests in a shorter time.

Which tests check directly for the virus?

Several laboratory procedures are used to test directly for the presence of HIV rather than for antibodies against it. Some of these methods involve exposing a person's blood serum to uninfected cells in the laboratory and testing to see whether the cells become infected. Other tests identify specific elements of the virus, such as proteins or enzymes. For example, some tests are designed to detect the enzyme reverse transcriptase, which is not found in healthy human cells but does exist in HIV. Tests that detect the presence of HIV itself are time consuming and expensive and require specialized lab facilities. They are most commonly used to help doctors determine the prognosis of an HIV-infected person. Knowing how much virus is in the bloodstream (viral load) provides information about the extent of HIV infection. Direct tests for HIV can also be used for diagnosing infants born to HIV-positive mothers. Because the mother's antibodies against HIV cross the placenta and reach the fetal bloodstream, babies born to HIV-positive women usually have antibodies against HIV even if they themselves are not infected. The result can be that the baby tests HIV positive because of its mother's antibodies not its own antibodies.

What is a PCR test?

Polymerase chain reaction (PCR) tests were first developed in the late 1980s and are used to diagnose many diseases. PCR tests allow small bits of genetic material to be amplified so that they can be identified as belonging to a specific type of virus. Because PCR can detect a small fragment of genetic material, it is a sensitive direct test for HIV.

What is a p24 antigen test?

The p24 antigen test is similar to the ELISA test, but instead of testing for antibodies against HIV, it tests for the presence of p24, a protein found in the core of HIV. The test is done on a person's blood plasma or other body tissue. HIV proteins, like p24, are found in the bloodstream at all stages of HIV infection, but they are most abundant during the first few weeks after a person gets infected and again at the later stages of infection.

Is there a saliva test for HIV?

Yes. One test for HIV uses a saliva sample instead of blood. The test uses similar laboratory procedures as are used in blood tests, and it too detects antibodies against HIV. Saliva tests are as reliable as blood tests but are not typically as available.

Is there a home HIV test kit?

Because some people have concerns about the confidentiality of getting tested for HIV by their doctor or a clinic, there is interest in at-home HIV test kits. Like at-home pregnancy tests, the home test for HIV allows a person access to private testing. The process for home testing usually involves the following:

- The person uses a small lancet included in the test kit to draw a few drops of blood collected by a piece of absorbent paper. This process is similar to that used for at-home cholesterol testing.
- Each piece of sample paper included in the test kit is tagged with a unique code number. This code allows the person to receive the test results without providing a name or any other identifying information.
- The dried blood drops are mailed to an HIV test laboratory.
- The blood is tested using the standard screening (ELISA) and confirming (Western blot) tests.
- The person telephones the lab and receives test results from a counselor.

Home testing for HIV is not, however, without its own concerns. Because having a positive HIV test can be emotionally devastating, home testing without the face-to-face counseling and guidance of a health care professional can leave someone on their own to deal with having HIV infection. Home testing can also mean that a person who tests positive for HIV is not connected to health care or referred to appropriate medical treatment. Nevertheless, home testing remains an option for getting tested for HIV.

When to Get Tested

Because HIV testing means that individuals may find out that they have a life-threatening disease, getting tested is a serious and personal decision. When people decide to get tested, they may have questions about the optimal time to get tested.

How long after possible exposure to HIV should people wait to get tested?

Before people get tested for HIV, they should wait until their body has time to produce antibodies against HIV. Tests done shortly after being exposed to HIV are not always accurate. Some people develop HIV antibodies as soon as 2 weeks after becoming infected, but most people exposed to HIV will have developed antibodies within 3 to 6 months after being infected. To be sure that HIV test results are accurate, people are advised to get tested twice, at least 3 months apart.

Can a person test HIV positive even after receiving a negative test result at an earlier time?

Having a negative HIV test result means that a person does not have antibodies against HIV at the time that their blood was drawn. During the time between HIV infection and the development of antibodies (an interval referred to as the *window period*), a person can test negative for HIV antibodies even though he or she is actually infected. When the test is repeated between 2 weeks and 6 months after infection occurred, the test can then detect antibodies.

If a person has two HIV negative tests in a row, can he or she still be infected?

People are usually advised to get tested again if they test HIV negative. A second HIV negative test result obtained 3 to 6 months after the first test assures that the original result was correct, provided that precautions were taken to avoid getting HIV after the initial HIV negative test result.

If someone tests HIV negative but is really positive because the test was done during the window period, can he or she transmit the virus to someone else?

Yes. A person who has HIV but tests negative during the window period can transmit the virus to others during sex or when sharing needles.

How often should a person get tested?

Whether and how often a person should get tested for HIV depend on many factors. For a person who has engaged in high-risk behavior but has not done so in the past 6 months, getting tested once is enough to indicate accurate HIV status. People with more recent risk behaviors should get tested at least twice to be sure their test results are accurate. People who continue to practice behaviors that place them at risk for HIV require repeated testing to learn if they become infected. Testing only tells a person if their body has produced antibodies against HIV at that point in time. Getting tested does not predict the future and does not protect people from getting infected.

Does getting tested for HIV help prevent AIDS?

The HIV antibody test is a medical diagnostic test. Just as a chest X-ray cannot prevent lung disease, HIV testing does not prevent AIDS. However, HIV testing should always occur within the context of at least a pretest and posttest counseling session. HIV counseling in conjunction with testing is intended to assist people in reducing their HIV risk behaviors and to help prevent AIDS.

What is repeat testing?

Repeat testing usually refers to getting tested every so often, perhaps every 3 or 6 months, over an extended time. Although a single repeated test is suggested when a person tests HIV negative to confirm the accuracy of the result, repeat testing over a longer period is not necessary to confirm a negative result. People who get tested repeatedly may be practicing risky behaviors between tests, and they are simply monitoring whether they have yet become HIV positive.

Are HIV tests done at the same time as tests for other STDs, like gonorrhea and syphilis?

It is possible to get tested for HIV at the same time as tests for other sexually transmitted diseases (STDs). Most clinics that diagnose and treat other STDs also offer HIV testing. However, the HIV test cannot be done as a part of a routine medical examination because a person's informed consent is needed before HIV testing.

The Testing Experience

Getting tested for HIV means taking the risk of finding out that one has a life-threatening disease. People who get tested usually have concerns about their own personal risk for infection and experience anxiety while waiting for their test results.

What happens during HIV testing?

The standard steps involved in going for HIV antibody testing are illustrated in Exhibit 6.1 and involve the following:

EXHIBIT 6.1. The HIV Testing Experience

Event	*What to expect*
Decision to get tested	Personal decision Weigh the pros and cons
Find a comfortable and affordable testing service	Consider confidentiality of results, low or no cost, good reputation for counseling, sensitivity
Pretest counseling	Discussion of the test and possible results Risk reduction strategies Personal risk assessment
Blood is drawn and sent to the lab	Blood drawn in vials like for other blood tests
Waiting period	Typically 1 to 2 weeks for analyses to be completed and results delivered
Notification of test results and posttest counseling	Results are given in privacy Referrals to services Continued risk reduction
Follow-up and referral	HIV-positive and HIV-negative people are provided with referrals to additional services

- The person provides written informed consent in the presence of a health care professional who explains what the HIV test is and what its results mean. In most situations, a person cannot be tested for HIV without giving informed consent.

- The person receives pretest counseling that usually lasts 5 to 30 minutes. Counseling includes an explanation of the test, discussions of what the limits of confidentiality are (unless the test is anonymous), personalized risk counseling to help a person gauge what the past risks have been, and exploration of individual concerns about the possibility of testing positive and the emotional aftermath of testing positive or negative.
- The test procedure itself involves drawing blood from the arm. This part of the test is very much like other blood tests.
- The blood sample is sent for laboratory analysis.
- Posttest result notification and counseling usually occur about 2 weeks after the initial visit. A counselor tells the person the test result and assists the person in coping and taking preventive action in the future.

Counseling is an important part of HIV testing, both before taking the test and after notification of results. Some settings are better able to offer pretest and posttest counseling than others. It is important to know which testing sites offer counseling when deciding where to get tested.

Can a couple go for testing together?

Yes. Couples can get tested together and receive counseling together or separately. The support of a friend or partner during testing can be important. Receiving results together is also possible, but it requires a willingness to share. Clinics differ in how they handle couples getting tested. For some couples, getting tested together can help reduce the stress of the testing experience, whereas for others testing could cause stress in the relationship. HIV testing counselors can help couples decide whether to get tested together or separately.

How much does it cost to get tested?

The cost of HIV testing varies from doctor to doctor and clinic to clinic. Office charges and additional lab costs vary greatly. However, testing can also be obtained completely free. Local health departments, STD clinics, and AIDS service organizations regularly offer free HIV testing. Information about where free testing is available can be obtained from state and local AIDS hotlines (see Appendix E), health departments, and the American Red Cross.

Where can a person get tested?

HIV testing is available from private doctors, clinics, health departments, and AIDS organizations. When finding a place to get tested, it is important to ask questions about the privacy of test results, the cost of testing, and the availability of counseling and referral services.

How long does it take to get test results?

The standard HIV test involves waiting between drawing blood and notification of results. Depending on how busy the clinic or lab is, it generally takes about 2 weeks for a person to get results from a standard HIV antibody test.

What is a rapid HIV test?

A rapid test allows for same-day test result notification. Rapid testing includes the same pretest, laboratory processes, and posttest counseling that is involved in standard testing. The technology for rapid testing is being developed and requires governmental approval before it can become available.

HIV Test Results

After blood is tested for HIV antibodies, the results are sent back to the clinic. Although people in the past had received test results by mail or telephone, the importance of counseling as a part of receiving results is now accepted as a fact. The possible results of an HIV antibody test result are shown in Exhibit 6.2.

What does a positive test result mean?

When a person tests HIV positive, it means that a sufficient amount of HIV antibodies were detected in their blood to allow a diagnosis of HIV infection. For a test to be positive, the following must occur:

EXHIBIT 6.2. HIV Antibody Test Results

Test result	*Explanation*
HIV negative	The ELISA test was nonreactive to HIV antibodies. Conclusion: Person has not developed antibodies against HIV.
HIV positive	The ELISA test reacted to HIV antibodies and was repeated and reacted again. Positive ELISA tests confirmed by Western blot test. Conclusion: Person has been exposed to and has developed antibodies against HIV.
Inconclusive	Possibly ELISA tests were positive but not confirmed by Western blot test, or ELISA tests were positive and Western blot only reacted to one element of HIV. Conclusion: Either the test mistook other antibodies for HIV antibodies or the person was seroconverting to HIV.
False positive	Rare incorrect positive test result Occurs with laboratory errors, or from reaction to non-HIV antibodies
False negative	Rare incorrect negative test result Can occur when person is tested during HIV antibody window period

- The ELISA screening test must be positive for HIV antibodies.
- The ELISA test must be repeated to assure that the first one was correct.

- ELISA results must be confirmed by the more specific Western blot test.

What does a negative test result mean?

A negative HIV test result means that the person's blood did not have detectable HIV antibodies. Because the ELISA test is sensitive to HIV antibodies, it is not necessary to repeat or confirm negative test results. A negative HIV antibody test does not mean that a person is not HIV infected but rather that they have not produced antibodies against HIV. A person can be infected for too short a time, usually no longer than 3 to 6 months, and has not yet produced antibodies at the time of testing.

What does it mean if a person's HIV test is nonreactive?

A *nonreactive* test result is another name for a negative test result—it means that the person's blood did not react in the testing procedure, which is another way of saying that the test did not detect HIV antibodies.

What is an inconclusive or undetermined test result?

In addition to receiving either a positive or negative result, a third possible outcome from an HIV antibody test is an indeterminate result, neither conclusively positive nor negative. Indeterminate HIV test results usually occur when the ELISA test is positive but the two required specific antibodies are not detected by the Western blot test. Inconclusive HIV test results can occur when the test is conducted during the antibody window period when a person is infected with HIV but is still in the process of developing antibodies. A person with an inconclusive test result should be retested again between 3 and 6 months later.

What is a false-positive test result?

A false-positive result occurs when the tests say that a person does have a disease when in fact he or she really does not have the disease. In HIV testing, false positives mean that a person's test results show HIV when in fact it is not present. Fortunately, false-positive HIV test results are rare because HIV testing is done in several steps, which include repeating a sensitive screening test and then subjecting the blood to a confirming test. False positives occur when both the ELISA and Western blot tests react to antibodies that are confused with HIV antibodies. Although it is more common for ELISA tests to obtain false-positive results, false-positive Western blot tests can also occur. Figure 6.1 illustrates the relationship between the window period and HIV test results.

What is a false-negative test result?

A false-negative result occurs when a test shows that a person does not have a disease when in fact he or

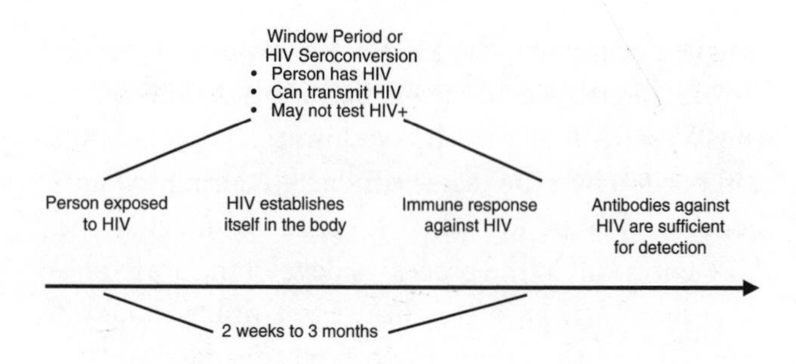

FIGURE 6.1. Relationship between the window period for developing HIV antibodies and HIV test results.

she really does. In the case of HIV infection, this means that a person's blood did not show HIV antibodies on the ELISA screening test even though the person really is infected. False-negative HIV tests are more frequent than false positives. The most common cause of a false-negative HIV test result is when a person gets tested during the window period between infection and the production of antibodies.

Is it possible for a person to test HIV negative and still have symptoms of HIV infection?

The earliest signs of HIV include an acute reaction to the infection. Most of these symptoms appear like other viral infections, including fatigue, low-grade fever, and swollen glands, and occur around the same time that the body is producing antibodies against the virus. Therefore, for a brief time during seroconversion a person can test negative for HIV antibodies and yet have some of the earliest symptoms of infection.

How accurate is HIV testing?

HIV antibody testing is among the most accurate diagnostic tests in medicine. The procedures used for HIV testing are 99% accurate, and confirmatory tests are more than 99% correct at pinpointing which antibodies have been produced.

Are test results from different labs equally accurate?

Every lab has its own standards, backlogs, and quality assurance procedures. Medical labs in the United States that test for HIV antibodies use similar procedures and have similar standards. Thus, HIV tests are usually equally reliable from different labs. Still, there is always a possibility that a laboratory has made an error. Whenever a test result is in doubt, a person should get retested.

Are certain people more likely to have inaccurate HIV test results?

Although rare, false positives are more likely in people who have had blood transfusions and in women who have had children. Also, recent vaccination for other illnesses, like the flu or hepatitis, can result in an inconclusive HIV test result. These experiences increase the chance for a false-positive result because cross-reacting antibodies have been produced in response to the blood transfusions, pregnancies, and vaccinations.

Privacy of HIV Testing

More than many other medical diagnoses, getting tested for HIV raises concerns about privacy. Knowledge that individuals have HIV infection can put them at risk for discrimination and prejudice. The simple fact of getting tested for HIV can lead to erroneous conclusions about the person being gay, promiscuous, or a drug user. These and other concerns have made privacy a priority for people who get tested for HIV.

When is testing confidential?

Like all aspects of a doctor–patient relationship, HIV testing ordered by private physicians and medical clinics remains a part of confidential medical records. However, like other medical information, HIV test results can be subject to release. For example, it is sometimes necessary to give employers and insurance companies permission to access confidential medical records. Medical information is therefore confidential but can be made available under special circumstances.

What is anonymous testing?

People who get tested anonymously never give their name as part of the test. Instead, their blood vial is coded with a number that is used for obtaining results. Returning for results involves seeing a counselor who has a record of test results matched to code numbers. Regardless of whether the result is positive or negative, people who are tested anonymously cannot be connected to their test results. Anonymous testing assures not only that test results are private, but also that the person's identity is not recorded. See Exhibit 6.3 for the differences between confidential and anonymous HIV antibody testing.

EXHIBIT 6.3. Confidential Versus Anonymous HIV Testing

Confidential	*Anonymous*
Name is given at testing site.	Name is not given to the testing site—tests are number coded.
Test results are placed in a medical record.	There is no medical record of the result.
People who test positive can be located and informed of their test results.	People who test positive cannot be located and informed of their result.
State health department is provided with test result.	State health department is provided with test result.
Positive test results can be used to notify health departments, past sex partners, health care providers.	Positive test results cannot be connected to the person who was tested.

Can a person be tested without being informed that the test is being done?

HIV testing requires that a person be informed about the test and what the results mean and that they give their consent to be tested. Patients have the right to prior informed consent and should be aware that they are being tested before testing. There are situations, however, when people can be tested without providing consent. Laws governing HIV testing vary from state to state. Situations where testing is mandatory and may supercede the requirement for informed consent include the following:

- The military provides its own blood supply, and testing is used to protect against transmission through transfusion as well as other situations that involve exposure to blood.
- Some municipalities require police and firefighters to get tested.
- Prison inmates and people arrested for prostitution are required to be tested in some states.
- Emergency room patients in some hospitals are tested as a matter of routine screening.
- Health care workers who practice invasive procedures can be required to get tested.

When minors are tested, do their parents have to give consent and be informed of the results?

HIV testing done by a clinic or private doctor is like other medical tests that are subject to requirements for parental consent for treatment and informing parents of test results. However, some states allow minors to be tested without consent, and states that provide anonymous testing may offer these services to teenagers.

Do insurance companies find out HIV test results?

It is common for insurance companies to require a physical examination and comprehensive health history prior to providing health, hospitalization, or life insurance. Many insurance companies have added HIV testing to the tests they routinely require. It became well known that insurance companies test for HIV when basketball star Magic Johnson tested HIV positive as a result of a medical exam for insurance purposes.

Is the HIV test done as part of routine blood work?

HIV testing can be done as part of annual physicals or other routine checkups. HIV testing is not, however, usually done without the person being informed.

Is HIV testing done as part of routine prenatal screening?

Because HIV can pass through the placenta to infect the fetus, HIV testing of women early in pregnancy is considered important. Hence, women are informed of the potential risks of HIV transmission. Studies show that using anti-HIV medications can significantly reduce the risks of infecting the fetus. There is a debate over whether HIV testing should be required as part of prenatal care or if pregnant women should retain their right to choose HIV testing. However, most women who are offered voluntary HIV testing accept it as part of their prenatal care. It is now recommended that all pregnant women be screened for HIV.

Are people required to get tested before they get married?

Some states require couples to get tested for HIV before they are granted marriage licenses. States often require health screening before marriage, such as tests for syphilis and blood type compatibility. The main idea behind premarital blood tests is to prevent the spread of disease and identify the risk of birth defects.

Who must know when a person tests HIV positive?

Every state requires doctors, hospitals, and other medical professionals to report AIDS diagnoses to state health departments for the purpose of tracking the course of the epidemic. Laws regarding reporting of HIV antibody test results, however, vary from state to state. Some states require that the names of people who test HIV positive be reported to state health authorities. Other states report HIV infection cases anonymously. Still other states do not require any reporting of HIV-positive test results. When cases are reported by name, health authorities may seek to identify and notify any person who could be at risk of having been infected. The only people who must know if a person has tested HIV positive are past sex and injection drug-equipment-sharing partners who may have been infected.

Can a person find out the test results of former sex partners?

HIV test results are either confidential or anonymous, so it not possible for someone to find out another person's test results. People who believe that they may have been exposed to the virus may wish to get tested. However, no one has the right to access another person's medical records without permission or a court order. Even when health authorities notify people that they may have been exposed to HIV, the name of the person who may have infected them is not provided.

Deciding to Get Tested

There are many good reasons to get tested for HIV, and there are many good reasons why a person would not want to get tested. Individuals must decide for themselves about getting tested. The decision involves their mental preparedness for learning they have the virus that causes AIDS, their financial situation, health insurance, relationship status, employment, family relationships, and other factors.

Should everybody get tested?

Each individual must decide whether to get tested for HIV. Many people who have not been at high risk for HIV still choose to be tested. People who have engaged in high-risk activities, those most likely to be infected, often feel anxious and may avoid getting tested. First and foremost, HIV testing is an individual decision, and it is not possible to say who should and who should not get tested.

What are the benefits of getting tested?

HIV testing offers a person the potential benefits of

- making informed decisions to protect sex partners,
- obtaining the relief that comes with knowing whether one has the virus,
- assuring those who test HIV negative that they have not yet been infected and that they can take precautions to keep from getting the virus,
- getting access to medical treatments that help an HIV-positive person stay healthy, and
- informing women whether they could transmit HIV during pregnancy.

Why would a person avoid getting tested?

People may choose not to get tested for HIV for the following reasons:

- They fear they cannot cope with a positive HIV test result.

- They would have to face past behaviors that they would rather forget.
- They worry that test results may not be confidential.
- They believe that it doesn't matter whether they have the virus, because there is no cure.
- They fear being labeled a high-risk person.
- They are concerned that they may face AIDS discrimination and prejudice.

Why should people get tested if they are in a long-term relationship?

Being in a long-term, exclusive relationship reduces a person's risk of getting the virus in the future. However, HIV testing tells a person if they have the virus from past behavior. Being in a committed relationship can only protect people from getting HIV if both partners do not already have the virus.

What can make testing less frightening?

People should not be tested for HIV unless they are mentally prepared. HIV testing usually includes counseling for this very reason. Before getting tested, people should consider

- what past behaviors may have placed them at risk,
- the meaning of positive and negative test results,
- who they can rely on for support in case they test HIV positive,

- their plan of action if the result is positive, and
- their own personal coping strategies for receiving either a positive or negative test result.

Talking with a health professional ahead of time about testing and having thought through the decision to get tested can make the experience less frightening. Having a supportive person or friend know about the test can help build a safety net and perhaps make getting tested less frightening.

SUMMARY

HIV testing is a personal decision. Many testing options are available to make testing more accessible. Testing can either be confidential, in which there is a medical record of the test, or anonymous, in which the person's name is not recorded. Testing can also have a cost for the service or testing may be free. HIV testing is among the most accurate of medical tests, but it is not a means of prevention; getting tested does not substitute for practicing safer sex and other preventive behaviors.

7

How Are People With AIDS Cared For?

AIDS is a devastating disease. People with HIV infection require a considerable amount of medical care, and HIV takes a toll that goes well beyond the immune system. Unlike other life-threatening diseases, such as cancer, HIV infection lasts for years without symptoms, and there is only cautious hope for a complete cure. People living with HIV require a great deal of medical and emotional care over the long course of their HIV infection.

Treatments for HIV and AIDS

Since AIDS was first identified in 1981, there have been thousands of experimental treatments for HIV. But until the mid-1990s there were only a few treatments available to people living with HIV. The treatment of HIV infection underwent a revolution in 1996 when new and highly effective medications were introduced. Medical treatments for HIV infection generally either target HIV itself or treat the diseases that result after HIV has disabled the immune system.

What treatments are available for HIV infection?

Exhibit 7.1 summarizes the major classes of medications that are used for treating HIV infection. The first drug approved for the treatment of HIV infection

EXHIBIT 7.1. Major Classes of Anti-HIV Medications

Drug class	*Drug brand (generic) name*
Single combination nucleoside reverse transcriptase inhibitors (NRTI)	Epivir (lamivudine, 3TC) Hivid (zalcitabine ddC) Retrovir (zidovudine AZT/ZDV) Videx (didanosine ddl) Zerit (stavudine d4T) Ziagen (abacavir sulfate)
Multiple NRTI	Trizivir (abacavir) Combivir
Nucleotide reverse transcriptase inhibitor	Viread (tenofovir)
Non-NRTI	Rescriptor (delavirdine mesylate) Sustiva (efavirenz) Viramune (nevirapine)
Protease inhibitors	Agenerase (amprenavir) Crixivan (indinavir sulfate) Fortovase (saquinavir) Invirase (saquinavir mesylate) Kaletra (lopinavir/ritonavir) Norvir (ritonavir) Viracept (nelfinavir mesylate)

Note. This list was complete when this book was published, but new HIV medications are rapidly becoming available, so the list is now likely to be incomplete.

was AZT (also called zidovudine), a drug that was originally developed in the 1960s to treat viral infections in animals. AZT is a medication that specifically targets the activity of retroviruses, including HIV. AZT interferes with the process by which HIV reproduces itself. The specific target of AZT is reverse transcriptase, an enzyme that is necessary for the replication of HIV. Treatment with AZT decreases the replication activity of HIV, increases the number of T-helper lymphocyte cells, reduces the illnesses that people with HIV are vulnerable to, and improves the general health of people infected with HIV. People who take AZT develop AIDS later and survive longer than people who are not treated.

In addition to AZT, other anti-HIV drugs also interfere with reverse transcriptase, including dideoxycytidine (ddC), dideoxyinosine (ddI), 3′-deoxythymidine-2′-ene (d4T), and Combivir and abacavir (combination nucleoside reverse transcriptase inhibitors). These drugs all belong to the family of nucleoside reverse transcriptase inhibitors—they insert a substitute molecule in the chain that builds the enzyme reverse transcriptase so that it will not work. Another important class of anti-HIV medications consists of the non-nucleoside reverse transcriptase inhibitors, including delavirdine, nevirapine, and efavirenz. The non-nucleoside reverse transcriptase inhibitors act by attaching themselves to reverse transcriptase to keep it from synthesizing HIV RNA into DNA. In addition, protease inhibitor medications (such as indinavir, ritonavir, nelfinavir, and saquinavir) target a very different HIV enzyme: protease. These drugs are usually used in combinations because they are capable of effectively hitting HIV at multiple points in its replication cycle. Other classes of medications that target additional enzymes, such as integrase, provide the promise of even further slowing the advance of HIV infection.

How do treatments for HIV work?

Treatments for HIV do not eliminate the virus from the body. Instead, they work to stop or slow down the reproduction of HIV. Different drugs have different ways of working, depending on the point of the HIV cycle at which they take action. For example, reverse transcriptase inhibitors block the enzyme responsible for replicating HIV genetic material. In contrast, protease inhibitors block the enzyme that plays a role in repackaging new virus particles.

What are combination therapies?

For HIV infection, *combination therapy* refers to the use of multiple medications that target different points of the HIV replication cycle to slow the virus down. It is common for three drugs to be used in combination, one of which is usually a protease inhibitor. However, combination therapy may include as few as two and as many as five or six different drugs.

What is HAART?

HAART stands for highly active anti-retroviral therapy, a name that is commonly used to refer to HIV combination therapies that include a protease inhibitor.

How do doctors know whether HIV treatments are working?

The goal of anti-HIV medications is to slow the progression of HIV infection by reducing the amount of viral replication. Doctors monitor the amount of HIV genetic material circulating in blood plasma, or viral load, as a means of observing the effects of HIV treatments. When a viral load drops, it is a marker for the effects of anti-HIV medications, and treatment is successful when viral load is suppressed to levels below detection. In addition, effective HIV treatment may be reflected in CD4 cell counts, indicating improvement in immune functioning.

Is it true that mixing anti-HIV medications with street drugs could kill you?

Yes. Some deaths have been associated with taking certain street drugs while taking anti-HIV therapies. Even the use of alcohol can have adverse interactions with some HIV treatments. People who are taking anti-HIV medications should always ask their doctor before using any nonprescription drugs.

What does it mean to adhere to HIV medications?

HIV treatments require people to take these drugs on schedule, as directed, and to never miss a dose. In some cases this can mean taking dozens of pills several times a day, some with meals and some without meals. For many people with HIV, the demand for close medication adherence is a significant challenge. Unlike nearly any other treatment of a chronic illness, HIV treatments demand close adherence to the prescribed dose because HIV can rapidly evade treatments when medication levels are relaxed. HIV can quickly develop resistance to treatments, ultimately rendering the medications ineffective.

What is a drug holiday?

A *drug holiday* is when a person ceases all medications. In some cases, doctors may suggest stopping treatment prior to switching to a new drug or combination of drugs. It is generally a bad idea for people on anti-HIV medications to stop treatment on their own without their doctor knowing because HIV can rapidly develop resistance to medications that are stopped and restarted.

What is treatment resistance?

Treatment *resistance* occurs when a virus (or bacteria or other disease-causing agent) develops immunity to a medication or medications. This occurs when a genetic selection or mutation inhibits specific treatment effects. In the case of HIV, the virus can rapidly mutate into treatment-resistant strains. Some HIV treatment-resistant strains are unaffected by multiple classes of HIV medications. Treatment-resistant strains of HIV can be transmitted to others who are then unlikely to benefit from available HIV treatments.

What is the difference between treatments for HIV and treatments for AIDS?

HIV treatments directly target HIV. Treatments for AIDS, and the diseases that occur when the immune system breaks down, attack other viruses, fungi, bacteria, and parasites but do not treat HIV infection itself. Treatments for AIDS-related opportunistic illnesses can cure infections and cancers that invade the body when the immune system has collapsed. Prevention and treatment of opportunistic illnesses is an important aspect of treating people with AIDS and has extended the lives of many AIDS patients.

How effective are HIV medications?

Combination therapies used in treating HIV infection can be very effective in suppressing the replication activity of HIV and extending the lives of people living with HIV/AIDS. Today's HIV treatments are given in smaller doses than in the early days of AIDS, and several drugs within several classes of medications are used in combination. Currently available treatments have brought hope for further controlling the course of HIV infection.

What are the side effects of anti-HIV medications?

People who take anti-HIV medications do so with the understanding that there are several possible side effects. Some people experience headaches, sleeping problems, nausea, vomiting, diarrhea, fatigue, skin rashes, aches and pains, and fever. Fortunately, side effects of anti-HIV medications often do not last long and can usually be resolved. It is essential that people who experience side effects of their HIV treatments inform their doctor and not stop taking their medications on their own.

What is lipodystrophy?

Lipodystrophy refers to changes in fat deposits, including loss of fatty tissue in the face and other body areas. Lipodystrophy can result as a side effect of some protease inhibitors. Changes in appearance that result from lipodystrophy can be emotionally difficult for people to handle.

What are alternative and complementary therapies?

Most medications prescribed by doctors for treating HIV infection and opportunistic illnesses are considered traditional or standard treatments. These medications must go through a stringent process of government approval to ensure their safety and effectiveness before they are made available. Treatments that are not yet formally approved constitute one type of nontraditional care. Some people choose nontraditional treatments instead of standard care, whereas others combine both traditional and nontraditional therapies. Nontraditional approaches are therefore often referred to as *complementary treatments*. Some complementary treatments can reduce levels of anti-HIV medications, thereby reducing their effectiveness. It is therefore important to consult a doctor or pharmacist before adding a complementary treatment to standard anti-HIV medications.

How can you tell if an advertised treatment is legitimate or a scam?

People with chronic illnesses can be desperate for a cure or effective treatment. For example, articles, books, and Web sites proclaim ozone treatments, blood-heating treatments, removal of parasites, and herbs as cures for AIDS. These claims often include testimonials from doctors or successfully treated patients. As a general rule, if a treatment sounds too good to be true it probably is. Asking a credible physician who treats HIV or other medical professional is a good way to check out the credibility of an advertised treatment.

What are AIDS clinical trials, and how can people find out about them?

AIDS clinical trials are a group of research programs, conducted by the National Institute for Allergies and Infectious Diseases of the National Institutes of Health and by drug companies, that are designed to test new treatments. People who enroll in a clinical trial agree to participate in research to help find better ways to treat people with HIV infection. Patients in clinical trials usually receive one type or dose of a treatment being tested against a different type or dose of treatment. Because clinical trials are carefully controlled research studies, people usually have to meet specific health criteria to be accepted. For more information about AIDS clinical trials, contact some of the clinical trials Web sites included in Appendix E.

Are researchers any closer to a cure for HIV?

It is unclear whether treatments that rid the body of HIV will ever be found. However, even if there is never a "silver bullet" that cures HIV infection, there are two reasons for hope. First, it is possible to prevent HIV infection from ever happening by taking action against the virus entering the body. Second, for people who are already infected, new treatments continue to be developed that are shown to slow the virus. Also impressive are the advances in treatments for the secondary infections and cancers that threaten people with damaged immune systems. Although HIV infection may never be curable, there is hope that HIV will continue to become a completely manageable chronic illness, perhaps like diabetes. The hope for managing HIV as a chronic illness is realistic and perhaps even within grasp.

Is there more hope for people with HIV infection today?

Yes. People with HIV are living longer today than ever before, and it is expected that in the future they will live even longer. The number of people dying of AIDS has slowed dramatically because of breakthroughs in medical treatments for HIV and medications for treating AIDS-related diseases. By slowing down the virus and preventing illness, there is much more hope for people infected with HIV today than there was in the past, and there is more hope for the future.

FINDING HELP

In the early days of the AIDS epidemic, people who were infected with HIV had few places to turn to for help. Communities most affected by AIDS have responded to the epidemic by establishing grassroots organizations to meet the needs of people with HIV infection. Today, most major cities and surrounding areas have service providers who specialize in helping people with HIV and AIDS.

Where can a person get help with medication adherence?

Taking medications for HIV infection on schedule and without missing a dose is one of the greatest challenges facing people living with HIV. Fortunately, there is help. Pillboxes that allocate daily doses and timers and alarms can serve as reminders for taking medications. Developing a routine for taking medications that becomes part of daily living is another common strategy for sticking to HIV treatments. Doctors who prescribe anti-HIV medications often have patient assistance materials and resources available from drug companies. It is also often beneficial to share ideas and strategies with other people living with HIV who are also taking anti-HIV medications, such as at AIDS support organizations or support groups.

What kind of services can help people stay home and out of the hospital or nursing home after they have developed AIDS?

People with AIDS require specialized medical care, particularly from specialists in infectious diseases. Services are available to help people with chronic illnesses remain at home and stay out of the hospital. Home nursing care and other health services are often available through home health agencies. AIDS service organizations also provide supportive services for people with AIDS. Volunteers serve as buddies to people with AIDS and help out by providing support and personal assistance. Buddies can also help prepare meals and run errands. Meal delivery and homemaker services are also available. Helpers are often assembled into teams to assure that a person's needs are met. AIDS service organizations can usually help access support services through a case management system. Together, coordinated efforts can serve to give people with AIDS enough support to stay at home as long as they wish.

What is a hospice, and how can it help people with AIDS?

Hospice is an approach to caring for people who are terminally ill when their recovery is unlikely and their life expectancy is stated in terms of months or weeks. Hospice care emphasizes quality rather than quantity of life. Holistic approaches to controlling pain, including psychological and spiritual pain, are embraced by hospice care. Family members and others in a person's life are often included as a part of hospice care. Hospice emphasizes comfort and palliative care for patients with advanced terminal diseases when there is no hope for a cure. Hospice care therefore integrates psychological, social, and medical approaches to address the issues facing people with terminal illnesses. People with AIDS may receive care from a general hospice that cares for terminally ill people or from a hospice program that serves only people dying of AIDS.

Do only certain nursing homes accept people with AIDS?

People with AIDS often require specialized care that is not available from many nursing homes or other long-term care facilities. At the later stages of AIDS, people may have needs that require convalescent care. For this reason, only specialty nursing homes provide care to people with AIDS.

Are some doctors better able to care for AIDS patients than others?

Yes. Because AIDS is caused by a virus and is the result of the body's inability to defend itself, infectious disease specialists and immunologists are best trained to deal with HIV patients. Infectious disease doctors are trained in methods for diagnosing and treating AIDS-related diseases. Immunologists are experts in the body's immune system, the target of HIV. Most doctors who provide primary care to people with HIV infection and AIDS are specialists in infectious diseases or immunology.

How can people with HIV find a dentist who will treat them?

Dentists cannot ethically turn a patient away because they have HIV infection. Dentists will often ask their patients if they have tested positive for HIV, as a part of a general medical history. Because many dental procedures by their very nature are invasive and expose dentists to a patient's blood, the American Dental Association and the Centers for Disease Control and Prevention (CDC) has established universal precautions to protect patients and dentists against infection.

How do people living with AIDS deal with euthanasia?

The last stages of AIDS, like those of many other terminal illnesses, can involve unbearable pain and suffering. Many people who are terminally ill therefore contemplate hastening their death when they see that the quality of their life has irreversibly declined. Of course, euthanasia raises numerous moral and ethical issues. Interest in euthanasia has increased in recent years with respect to AIDS and other illnesses that cause suffering and death in young people. Counseling can help people think through issues of hastening death. Hospice organizations and other services for individuals who are terminally ill often deal with euthanasia issues and can also help people face death.

Getting Support

People living with HIV have needs that go beyond those met by traditional medicine. Communities have responded in several ways to meet the emotional needs of people affected by AIDS.

Do people get counseling after they receive the news that they have HIV?

To receive federal funding for HIV antibody testing, the test process must include a pretest and posttest counseling session to ensure that a person understands what the test does and what its results mean. HIV posttest counseling for people who test HIV positive should assess the person's ability to cope with an HIV diagnosis, assess the person's support system, and include proper referrals for medical care. Unfortunately, many people who have tested HIV positive have not received the counseling they needed. It is therefore important to know what kinds of services are provided by a testing center before deciding to get tested.

Where can a person with HIV get counseling?

Most cities have counseling services available for people with HIV infection. It may be preferable to receive counseling from a professional who is knowledgeable about HIV and AIDS and who is familiar with the issues faced by people living with HIV infection. There are now counselors who have been trained to deal with the special issues of HIV infection. Information about how to go about finding a counselor with knowledge and understanding about AIDS can be obtained from the American Psychological Association and the National Association of Social Workers, both located at 750 First Street, NE, Washington, DC 20002. There are also self-help materials available for people coping with the stress of HIV infection. One example is a book by Michael Callen (described in the suggested reading section toward the end of this book) that provides one man's inspirational story of living and coping with AIDS. Help is also available in the form of relaxation and coping guidance.

What are AIDS support groups?

Support groups are a source of information and emotional support for people dealing with HIV infection. Support groups bring together people who have a common problem to share their experiences. A sense of shared meaning is one thing that support groups offer as a source of strength. There are many types of support, including

- tangible support, such as help with daily living chores and transportation;
- information support, including new knowledge and answers to questions; and
- emotional support, supplied by empathy and understanding.

Research has shown that many HIV-positive people who attend support groups appear to benefit from the experience.

Are there special support groups for gay men, women, and drug users?

Support groups are as different as the people who join them. Some support groups are formed for the purpose of bringing people with HIV together regardless of how they became infected with the virus. However, there are support groups for gay, bisexual, and heterosexual men; women; injection drug users; adolescents; and so forth. These groups work better for some people because they feel that special challenges face men, women, adolescents, and so on. On the other hand, some people feel they are part of an HIV-positive community first and foremost and are comfortable in a diverse group.

Are there AIDS support groups on the Internet?

Yes. HIV/AIDS support groups online are typically text-based, using instant messenger or chat communication systems. Online support groups have many advantages, including the convenience of attending a support group without leaving home, communicating with people with HIV from around the world, and being able to participate anonymously. Internet users should however use caution, check the credibility of the Web site, and be wary of purchasing health products that might be for sale online, using services that require payment, or attempting to meet members in person.

Help for Helpers

Caring for people with AIDS can be emotionally and physically demanding. The ups and downs and improvements and setbacks that come with AIDS can cause considerable stress. If having AIDS is like an emotional roller coaster, then the people who care for AIDS patients are along for the ride. Caregiver stress can lead to emotional burnout, making it difficult to continue providing high-level care.

Do community services assist people who care for AIDS patients?

Community-based AIDS organizations may offer a number of services to assist in the care of people with AIDS. Respite care for caregivers can offer relief from the demands of caring for someone with a terminal illness, assist with daily caregiving, and provide the psychological support of knowing that someone is there to help.

What resources are available to professional caregivers?

The potential for burnout is a concern for all professionals who treat people with any chronic illness; the risk is particularly high for AIDS caregivers. Unlike doctors who specialize in treating cancer, infectious disease physicians have historically been able to cure most of their patients. This has been particularly true since the advent of antibiotics and preventive vaccines. With HIV, however, infectious disease specialists now face an incurable disease that leads to multiple infections and other illnesses that are themselves difficult to treat. For these reasons, support groups, counseling, and informal support services have developed for professional caregivers, particularly in hospitals and clinics that serve a large number of people with AIDS.

Are there support groups for families and friends of people with HIV?

Yes. Support groups are often available for friends and family members of people living with HIV/AIDS. Community-based AIDS service organizations and infectious disease clinics are usually a source of these services.

Where can people get help after they have lost someone to AIDS?

People who have lost someone to a terminal illness often require support as they cope with the loss. Dealing with the loss of someone to AIDS is complicated by the stigmas that society has placed on this disease and by the fact that most people who die of AIDS are young. Counseling and support groups for the bereaved are often available through AIDS service agencies, religious organizations, clinics, and hospitals.

How can a person go about making a panel for the AIDS quilt?

The AIDS quilt has become an international symbol of remembrance for those who have died of AIDS. The quilt consists of panels, each of which represents an individual who died of AIDS. Friends and family of those who have died make panels that portray special qualities of the person and what his or her life meant. The AIDS quilt has grown to thousands of pieces, patched together into a blanket large enough to cover the grounds of entire city parks. Information about contributing to the quilt or about where it is displayed is available from The NAMES Project Foundation AIDS Memorial Quilt, P.O. Box 5552, Atlanta, GA 31107; (404) 688-5500; www.aidsquilt.org.

Staying Healthy

People living with HIV infection can take measures to be healthy. Avoiding things that could further reduce the immune system's ability to fight diseases can have positive health benefits. Increasing activities that bolster resistance against disease can also have health benefits.

What roles do nutrition and exercise play in staying healthy?

Eating properly and keeping fit offer the same health benefits to people who have HIV infection as they do to anyone. Eating nutritious food, getting plenty of rest, reducing stress, and exercising increase the body's ability to protect against and recover from illnesses. Although there is limited evidence that healthy living slows down HIV's destruction of the immune system, taking control of one's health can impede the diseases that strike when the immune system is damaged.

Is it important for people who have HIV infection not to smoke cigarettes and to avoid drinking alcohol?

Smoking and drinking both have adverse effects on the body's immune system and lower resistance against disease. In addition, smoking interferes with the healing processes of the lungs, which are particularly important for individuals with compromised immune systems. Drinking alcohol can also interact with HIV medications and interfere with their effects.

Should people who have HIV drink bottled water?

Water purification systems remove, among other things, bacteria and other parasites that can cause serious illness. Although drinking water in the United States is generally safe, water systems are not flawless. Tap water can contain parasites that cause little or no illness in people with healthy immune systems but can be devastating in people with HIV infection. Water purification systems can also fail and result in contaminated water. A case in point occurred in Milwaukee, Wisconsin, in the mid-1990s when the water system failed and resulted in an epidemic of cryptosporidium, a parasite that infects the intestines and causes chronic and debilitating diarrhea. Because there is no cure for cryptosporidium, it usually runs its course until the body builds up resistance. However, people with HIV infection are often unable to overcome cryptosporidium, and it can eventually lead to their death. Boiling tap water or drinking bottled water are the best ways for people with HIV infection to avoid waterborne parasites.

Can people with HIV do things to help rebuild their immune system?

A healthy immune system can be built up by improving general health through nutrition, exercise, rest, stress reduction, and so forth. Although these activities cannot reverse HIV's effects on the immune system, research shows that people with HIV experience health benefits to their immune system by taking care of their general health.

Can people with HIV have pet cats?

Cats can carry a parasite that causes illness for people with suppressed immune systems. Toxoplasmosis is an infection caused by the parasite *Toxoplasma gondii*, which is common in domestic cat feces. Toxoplasmosis can cause serious illness, including infections of the brain. Although toxoplasmosis responds well to treatment, it can leave irreversible damage. People with HIV infection are therefore advised not to have house cats, and they should be careful when gardening or doing other activities that could bring them into contact with cat feces.

Are people with AIDS put at risk if they are with someone who has a cold or the flu?

People with AIDS have seriously impaired immune systems, which makes recovery from any infection difficult. Although colds and the flu do not always become serious threats to people with early HIV infection, they can be difficult to get over and should be avoided, particularly after the immune system becomes damaged.

Can a person with HIV get vaccinated against the flu and other diseases?

People with HIV infection can usually be vaccinated against other diseases. Although the reactions that commonly occur after vaccination may be enhanced in people with suppressed immune systems, the CDC recommends vaccinations to prevent disease, and most people with HIV are at lower risk for side effects from the vaccine than they are from the infections themselves.

Summary

Community-based AIDS service organizations are often lifelines for people living with HIV infection and AIDS. These organizations often operate with minimal resources relative to the care they provide. Serving as a center point for AIDS care, AIDS service organizations offer a wide range of support that often includes transportation, legal services, case management, family support, financial assistance, meals, and social programs. Organizations often rely on volunteers, so volunteering for an AIDS organization is a great way to get involved.

8

What Are the Legal Aspects of AIDS?

AIDS has far-reaching effects on society as well as individuals, bringing countless challenges to the families, friends, and communities of people with AIDS. The social ramifications of AIDS have resulted in laws and policies directed at managing this complicated disease. This chapter addresses questions about laws and social policies affecting those who either are at risk or have become HIV infected.

Legal Issues

The AIDS epidemic raises legal issues for people at risk of contracting HIV, those already infected with the virus, and their friends and families. AIDS-related legal issues deal with insurance, employment, civil rights, privacy, family law, and other topics.

Does the law support individuals who wish to keep their HIV status confidential?

Yes. Like people with other medical conditions, there are laws that protect the confidentiality of persons living with HIV/AIDS. Laws that govern the limits of confidentiality, reporting of HIV-positive test results, and other aspects of privacy vary from state to state. However, confidentiality usually has limits and the law often determines these limits. Confidential medical information is often accessible by court order, and confidential information can be released when it is necessary to protect others.

Are the names of HIV-positive people reported to the government?

Medical personnel are often required to report the names of people with communicable diseases to state health departments for surveillance of the disease and attempts at public health control. However, because of the stigmas and discrimination often directed at people with AIDS, there has been opposition to divulging the names of HIV patients. Nevertheless, most states require confidential reporting of HIV infections to state health departments. Knowing the identities of people with HIV infection helps maintain accurate accounting of the rates of disease and also allows public health workers to identify potentially infected partners of people who test HIV positive.

Is it legal for a hospital or doctor to withhold treatment from a person who has HIV?

No. Discrimination by doctors against people with HIV/AIDS was common in the beginning of the AIDS crisis, particularly when the cause of AIDS was unknown. Fortunately, medical discrimination has become less likely as a result of advances made in our understanding of what HIV is, how the virus is transmitted, and how HIV causes AIDS. Human rights and antidiscrimination laws prohibit withholding access to care for people with disabling conditions, including HIV and AIDS. In addition, the Americans with Disabilities Act (ADA), signed into law in 1990, protects people with HIV from being denied access to public services, including medical care. Medical professionals may refer patients who have HIV to specialists if they are not trained to deal with this complex disease. However, such referrals must be based on the needs of the patient. Thus, both laws and professional ethics protect AIDS patients against medical discrimination.

Are there laws that require people to get tested if they might have infected someone with HIV?

With rare exceptions, people cannot be forced to have an HIV antibody test. Public health officials can advise and encourage people who have been sexually involved with, or shared injection needles with, someone who has HIV to get tested. HIV testing is a medical diagnostic test, so people have the right to choose whether they want to be tested. There are, however, exceptions to this rule. For example, some states have mandatory HIV testing for prison inmates because of the potential for spreading the virus in prisons through homosexual acts, sharing needles to inject drugs, or bloody fights. The U.S. military also requires its personnel to be periodically tested for HIV because the military serves as its own blood bank and because of the potential exposure to blood in combat situations. There is a great deal of debate about expanding mandated testing to people who are likely to have been at risk for HIV and to pregnant women, because such policies may infringe on personal rights and civil liberties.

Can people with AIDS get legal assistance in such matters as writing a will?

Yes. People infected with HIV often find themselves in need of legal services for things like wills, insurance, or discrimination. In addition to more general legal assistance, community-based AIDS service organizations often provide legal aid to their clients. In most cases, attorneys are asked to help people by answering legal questions, preparing legal documents, and writing a will.

Insurance

Catastrophic illnesses like AIDS carry extensive costs for medical care. Insurance is a major concern for many people infected with HIV. Insurance regulations vary greatly from state to state, which makes it difficult to provide answers to specific questions.

How long can a person who has HIV infection remain insured?

Unless it can be proven that a person was infected with HIV prior to the time their insurance began (making HIV a pre-existing condition for that person), people cannot lose their insurance coverage because they test HIV positive. However, a common problem that people with HIV infection encounter is that their insurance is tied to their employment, and so they often lose their insurance when they are no longer able to work. However, there are laws that protect a person's insurance benefits when they change or terminate their employment, particularly the Consolidated Omnibus Budget Reconciliation Act (COBRA) of 1985. Some insurance plans have options for continued coverage, but payment is still required.

What is the Ryan White Law?

Ryan White was an Indiana teenager who contracted HIV during treatment for hemophilia. Ryan White was discriminated against and not allowed to attend school because he was HIV positive. Because of his story of fighting the social stigmas of AIDS, his name is attached to the federal law that entitles HIV-positive people to medical care and social services. Public Law 101-381, the Ryan White Comprehensive AIDS Resources Emergency (CARE) Act, was signed into law in August 1990 and was reauthorized by President Bill Clinton in 1996. Between 1991 and 2000, more than

$6.4 billion in federal funds had been appropriated under the Ryan White CARE Act to serve hundreds of thousands of people living with HIV/AIDS in the United States.

Can a person with HIV infection qualify for Social Security benefits?

A person with HIV who develops AIDS may be eligible for Social Security benefits. In general, there are two programs: Social Security Disability Income (SSD) and Supplemental Security Income (SSI). SSD is like an insurance policy for those who have paid into the program sufficiently long enough through Social Security payroll deductions. These benefits become available to people who meet certain disability criteria, such as having an AIDS diagnosis and being unemployed. SSD benefits can include eligibility for Medicare, but there is usually a waiting period before coverage begins. SSI does not, however, draw from the nation's Social Security fund, does not require funds to have been paid in, and does not have a waiting period. SSI benefits usually include Medicaid and food stamps and are based on individual need. Details about these programs can be obtained from local Social Security offices and local AIDS service organizations.

Is there financial assistance that can help a person get prescriptions to treat HIV?

It is common for the treatment of advanced HIV and AIDS to require multiple expensive medications. Fortunately, public assistance programs offer help to people who cannot afford HIV treatments. For one, pharmaceutical companies may have patient assistance programs and reimbursement plans for people in need. Information about these programs can be obtained from the American Foundation for AIDS Research (1-800-39-AMFAR). Local AIDS organizations also have information about financial assistance, and some programs redispense unused medications for people in need.

Can an insurance company require a person to get tested for HIV infection?

Health and life insurance often requires a physical examination to test for medical conditions that exist before the coverage begins. Insurance companies have an interest in knowing what a person's health status is before underwriting an insurance policy. In some states, insurance companies can legally require a person to get tested for HIV on the basis of medical history or current health status, or if all people in the same risk class who are applying for the same type of insurance are required to get tested. In general, however, applicants are required to consent to the test.

Are there organizations that pay cash for a life insurance policy?

Yes. Life insurance policies have a cash value after a person has died. Clearly, however, money no longer does people any good after they die. Because people can live several years with AIDS and usually do so with a loss of income, there are options for selling life insurance benefits. People with AIDS who have valid life insurance policies can sell them to individuals or businesses that then become the beneficiaries of the policy. A percentage of the policy value is usually paid to policyholders, who receive the money for their own use while they are still alive.

Is there a place where people can turn to for help if their insurance company refuses to pay for health care?

Yes. Insurance companies have occasionally refused to pay for some HIV-related medical expenses. For example, they may refuse to cover people who are diagnosed with AIDS relatively soon after their insurance coverage starts because HIV infection takes years to cause AIDS. Coverage of certain treatments for HIV and AIDS has also been denied because they are considered experimental. Fortunately, AIDS service organizations offer assistance in dealing with insurance problems through case management and legal counsel. Also, state insurance commissioners can answer questions and receive complaints against insurance companies.

Rights of People With HIV/AIDS

Prejudice and discrimination against people living with HIV/AIDS remain significant problems. The groups most affected by AIDS in the United States include gay and bisexual men, drug abusers, and ethnic minorities, groups that have long been discriminated against. Worldwide, stigmas against AIDS account for acts of discrimination and violence against people living with HIV/AIDS. As experience with cancer, epilepsy, and other chronic illnesses has shown, fear breeds stigma and stigma leads to prejudice. AIDS stigma has spawned an epidemic of fear, prejudice, and discrimination against people living with HIV/AIDS.

Can people be held legally responsible if they infect others with HIV?

Some states have passed laws against knowingly placing others at risk for HIV infection. Several such cases have involved rape, prostitution, and consensual sexual relations, in which an HIV-positive person places someone at risk without disclosing his or her HIV status. Similar situations can arise when individuals with HIV risk exposing others to their blood in the workplace. Examples of state laws that criminalize exposing others to HIV are presented in Table 8.1. Thus, in some situations individuals who are HIV positive are held accountable for potentially infecting others.

TABLE 8.1. Selected State Criminal Statutes on the Transmission of HIV

State	*Statute*	*Text*
Arkansas	Ark. Code § 5–14-123	It is a Felony for a person who knows that he or she has tested positive for HIV to expose another to HIV through the transfer of blood or blood products by engaging in sexual intercourse, cunnilingus, fellatio, anal intercourse or any other intrusion into the genital or anal openings of another without first informing the other person of his or her positive status.
California	Health and Safety Code § 120291	Any person who exposes another to HIV through unprotected sexual activity or use of a hypodermic needle is guilty of a Felony, when the infected person knows he or she is infected, has not disclosed the information, and has acted with specific intent to infect the other person.
Florida	Fla. Stat. § 384.24	It is unlawful for any person who is infected with HIV, knowing of such infection and informed of the possibility of communicating the disease through sexual intercourse with any other person, to have sexual intercourse with any other person, unless such other person has been informed of the presence of the virus and has consented to the sexual intercourse.

Georgia	Ga. Cone Ann. § 16-5-60	Any person notified of their HIV-positive status, who exposes another through sexual activity; use of a hypodermic needle or syringe; or donates blood or other bodily fluids; or solicits or commits sexual acts for money, is guilty of a Felony.
Illinois	Ill. Ann. State Ch. § 5.12–16.2	A person commits criminal transmission of HIV when such person, knowing that he or she is infected with HIV: engages in intimate contact with another involving the exposure of one person to the body fluid of another, transfers, donates, or provides his or her blood, tissue, semen, organs, or other potentially infectious body fluid for transfusion, transplantation, insemination, or other administration to another; or dispenses, delivers, exchanges, or sells non-sterile intravenous, or intra-muscular drug paraphernalia.
Maryland	Health-Gen § 18-601.1	An individual who has HIV and knowingly transfers HIV to another individual is guilty of a Misdemeanor.
Nevada	Nev. Rev. Stat. Ann. § 201.205	Any person who has tested HIV-positive who knowingly or willfully acts in a manner intended to transmit HIV is guilty of a Felony.
New Jersey	N.J. Stat. Ann. § 2c:34-5	A person is guilty of a crime of the third degree when s/he commits an act of sexual penetration without informed consent of the other person knowing that s/he is infected with HIV.

Can people be fired from their jobs because they have HIV?

No. It is illegal for people who have HIV infection to be terminated from their employment because they have HIV, assuming that they are otherwise qualified and able to work. The ADA protects people with HIV from employment discrimination related to their condition. In fact, the law requires employers to make reasonable accommodations, such as flexible work hours or rest periods, to help disabled employees keep their jobs.

Can a person who has HIV be evicted from a rental house or apartment?

The Federal Fair Housing Amendments Act bans any form of housing discrimination against people with disabilities, including HIV/AIDS. This law was enacted after several years in which housing was denied to people with HIV or people stereotyped as being at high risk for HIV infection.

Can a business refuse to hire individuals with HIV infection?

No. The ADA applies to cases where a person with HIV experiences employment discrimination. The law allows HIV testing to be included as part of a physical exam required before starting a job, but the results cannot be made a condition of the employment. However, employees cannot be required to have the HIV test unless an employer can prove that it is necessary for the performance of their jobs.

Do people with HIV have to tell their doctor or dentist that they have the virus?

It is necessary that a doctor know a patient has HIV to provide that patient with adequate care. Doctors and dentists cannot deny treatment to people who have HIV infection. In addition, although all medical professionals should practice universal precautions against potential disease transmission, medical professionals have the right to be aware of potential risks they may be taking when performing invasive procedures on their patients. HIV infection is an important medical condition, and in most instances HIV status should be disclosed to medical care providers.

To whom does an HIV-positive person have to disclose his or her condition?

No laws govern when a person must be tested for HIV, and no laws direct people to disclose their HIV status unless they risk infecting others. People have a moral and ethical obligation, however, to inform others that could be exposed to the virus by having contact with their blood, semen, or vaginal fluids.

Are there countries that do not allow visitors who have HIV?

Several countries ban visits by people who are HIV positive. In the United States, the Immigration and Nationality Act states that "aliens who are infected with any dangerous contagious disease" should be prohibited from immigrating into the country. There have been several attempts to change this immigration law, but the ban remains in place and more countries are adding such laws in an effort to keep out people who have HIV. However, public health officials generally agree that prohibiting people with HIV infection from traveling has no significant effect on containing the virus and can interfere with access to experimental treatments and exchange of scientific information.

Do any countries quarantine people who have HIV infection?

Yes. Some countries quarantine people with HIV as an attempt to control the epidemic. For example, Cuba has had a quarantine policy to separate people who test HIV positive from the general population. Aside from the human rights violations that are obviously associated with quarantining people with HIV, quarantine is not an effective strategy for containing HIV.

Difficult Decisions and Ethical Dilemmas

Unlike questions about the biological, medical, legal, and even some of the social aspects of AIDS, there are few definitive answers to ethical and moral questions about AIDS. The following questions represent such issues. Only clarification of these issues, and not absolute answers, can be offered.

If a person knows that someone is HIV positive, does that person ever have the right to tell others?

Disclosing that someone else has HIV carries tremendous consequences. Certain situations can make disclosing someone's HIV status appear necessary, such as when a person is unknowingly being placed at risk by the actions of an infected person. However, even under these circumstances, disclosing that someone has HIV infection can be experienced as an act of betrayal and cause distress, discrimination, and other adverse conditions for the person living with HIV/AIDS.

What should a person do with the knowledge that someone who has HIV is knowingly spreading the virus to others?

There is no single course of action for individuals who believe that someone with HIV is putting others at risk. One option is to discuss the problem with the HIV-positive person. Beyond this, a person can only be advised to take whatever actions they feel necessary to help protect others against getting HIV. Contacting local health authorities or AIDS service organizations may help deal with these difficult situations.

Do people with HIV tell their prospective sex partners they have the virus?

Research shows that most people with HIV infection do tell their prospective sex partners that they have the virus. However, a minority of people living with HIV/AIDS do not always disclose that they are HIV positive to sex partners. It seems that the weaker the bond between the person with HIV and their partner, such as casual versus committed partners, the less likely they are to disclose. Few people with HIV keep their long-term sex partners unaware of their HIV status.

Where can people get help in dealing with disclosing their HIV status to others?

Disclosing HIV status is a significant challenge for many people living with HIV, especially people who have recently tested HIV positive. Counselors can help people in working through decisions whether to disclose and can advise them about the best way to disclose being HIV positive to others. It can also be helpful to hear others share their disclosure experiences and strategies for disclosure, and this is the kind of information shared in support groups.

Summary

AIDS affects society at many levels. The courts hear cases involving AIDS discrimination, privacy rights, and personal responsibility. Lawmakers contemplate mandatory HIV testing and placing restrictions on HIV-positive people who knowingly have unsafe sex. The expanding AIDS epidemic continues to raise many complex issues about how social structures can help prevent the spread of HIV. Still, personal responsibility, not public policy, remains the greatest hope for stopping AIDS.

9

How Is AIDS Prevented?

Perhaps the only good thing about AIDS is that it can be completely prevented by changing just a few behaviors. HIV enters the body when HIV-infected blood, semen, or vaginal fluids are transferred from one person to another. Preventing these fluids from entering the body eliminates all risks of HIV infection. Because almost all new cases of AIDS result from sexual intercourse and sharing needles to inject drugs, AIDS can be prevented by altering these behaviors.

Safer Sex

The term *safe sex* was coined in response to AIDS. Safe sex usually refers to sexual practices that protect a person from contracting or transmitting HIV and other sexually transmitted diseases (STDs). For sex to be truly safe, it must not carry any risk for transferring blood, semen, or vaginal fluids from one person to another. *Safer sex*, on the other hand, implies a reduction in risk, but not necessarily complete safety. See

EXHIBIT 9.1. Strategies for Effectively Reducing Sexual Risks for HIV and Other STDs

- *Objectively examine your own personal risk.* Any person who is either sexually active or shooting up drugs could be at risk for HIV. It is a person's behavior and the history of the sexual partners that place a person at risk. If you have ever had sex with someone who could have been exposed to HIV, then you may be at risk for HIV infection. Most people who have HIV infection do not even know it.
- *Consider whether you should seek counseling and testing.* The only way to know if you are HIV infected is to get tested for HIV. Prevention counseling is also available from many testing sites.
- *Talk with friends about HIV and AIDS.* Sharing ideas, concerns, and information with others is an important part of prevention. Let others know that AIDS is a threat and that each person can do something about the spread of HIV.

continued

Exhibit 9.1 for effective strategies for reducing the risk of HIV infection.

What is considered *safe sex*?

Safe sex means there is no risk of transmitting HIV or other STDs from person to person. In the simplest terms, safe sex does not allow mucous-membrane-to-mucous-membrane or blood-to-blood contact. It is sometimes mistakenly thought that using condoms is

EXHIBIT 9.1. *Continued*

- *Talk with sex partners about AIDS*. Get to know what your partners think about AIDS. Talk about getting tested together and about how condoms can be used as both birth control and caring for each other's health. Using male or female condoms expresses care and concern for a partner.
- *Know your own personal risky situations*. Sexual relationships can occur under all kinds of circumstances. Some people engage in risky behavior when they are depressed or stressed. Others do so when they are in love. For others, unprotected sex is linked to the use of alcohol or other drugs. The situations that create risk are usually apparent ahead of time and are called *risk triggers*. Knowing your own risk triggers allows you to make decisions to avoid risk.
- *Make condoms a part of satisfying sexual relations*. Most people who do not use condoms believe they interrupt the spontaneity of sex and decrease sexual pleasure. But many people have made condoms a part of meaningful and satisfying sexual relationships. Condoms can be made a part of sex by including both partners in their use. The stimulation provided by condoms can also be increased by using proper lubrication. There are many types of condoms, allowing for variety and novelty. Safer sex can be pleasurable for couples who are open to trying something new.

what is meant by safe sex. However, condoms occasionally leak or break, which makes them not completely safe. See Exhibit 9.2 for sexual acts that offer complete safety from transmitting HIV and other STDs.

EXHIBIT 9.2. Sexual Acts Safe From Transmitting HIV and Other STDs

Hugging and holding	Hugging does not allow person-to-person transfer of body fluids, so hugging, holding, and embracing are completely safe behaviors.
Kissing	Kissing, particularly deep kissing, does transfer saliva from person to person, but saliva has not been known to transmit HIV. Kissing is therefore a safe behavior.
Heavy petting	Petting usually means a lot of touching and deep kissing and is therefore a form of safe sex. It does not matter what body parts, including the genitals, are touched; HIV cannot enter the body through unbroken skin. Contact between mucous membranes and open sores or small cuts should be avoided. Under most circumstances, all sexual behaviors that do not involve the penis penetrating the vagina, anus, or mouth are considered safe.
Masturbation	Masturbation, manual stimulation of the genitals, usually with one's hand or perhaps an object, is usually thought of as a solitary sexual activity. However, manually stimulating or masturbating a partner is safe because blood, semen, and vaginal fluids do not enter a partner's body.
Foreplay	In some respects, safe sex is best described as foreplay. Think of all the things that people do together while having sex prior to the act of sexual intercourse.

What is *safer sex*?

Safer sex refers to practices that lower but do not remove the risks for HIV and other STDs. Examples of safer sex behaviors include oral sex where one partner's mouth comes in contact with the other partner's penis, but ejaculation does not occur in the mouth. The risk for HIV transmission in this sexual act is very low, but it cannot be considered risk free. The use of latex condoms during sexual intercourse significantly reduces the risk of HIV infection, but because condoms can leak and tear, this practice does not completely eliminate risk.

What is *negotiated safety*?

First popular in Australia and England, particularly in gay communities, *negotiated safety* encourages people to talk with their sex partners about what level of risk they are willing to take and to come to an agreement about practicing safer sex. For example, through conversation a couple may choose to practice unprotected oral sex but use a condom during all acts of vaginal and anal intercourse. As a couple they therefore agree to accept the relative risks of oral sex and the risks of condom failures. Negotiated safety assumes a certain level of relationship openness, comfort in discussing sex, and knowledge of what is safe and unsafe.

Is withdrawing the penis from the vagina or anus before ejaculation safer sex?

As many as 1 in 10 heterosexual couples use withdrawal or other forms of intercourse interruption to prevent pregnancy. Withdrawal of the penis prior to ejaculation does carry some risk for HIV infection (not to mention other STDs), although it lowers the risk somewhat. Unless condoms are used, the penis is exposed to vaginal fluids, and some fluids are discharged from the penis and enter the vagina or anus before ejaculation occurs. Pre-ejaculation fluids prepare the urethra for ejaculation and can carry sperm as well as viruses and bacteria that cause STDs. Thus, withdrawal practiced consistently and without mishap may be safer than taking no precautions at all—but probably not much safer.

Can fellatio be made safer?

Yes. Mouth-to-penis oral sex, or fellatio, is considered somewhat risky for transmitting HIV, although it is substantially less risky than vaginal and anal intercourse. Oral sex is a high-risk behavior, however, for many other STDs. Fellatio can be made safer either by using latex condoms or by avoiding contact between the mouth and head of the penis. Contact between the mouth and intact skin of the penis does not risk HIV transmission.

Why is a dental dam used?

A dental dam is a sheet of rubber or latex used to create a protective barrier during dental work. Dental dams are usually a few inches in size and square in shape. Because dental dams are made of latex, they can also provide a protective barrier when the mouth could come in contact with body fluids that may contain HIV, such as during cunnilingus (mouth–vagina contact) and rimming (oral–anal contact). Cunnilingus and rimming are relatively low-risk sexual acts with respect to HIV transmission; so placing a latex barrier between the mouth and vagina or anus reduces the chances of contracting HIV through these acts to nearly zero.

Can birth control methods also prevent HIV?

Male and female condoms are the only methods that effectively prevent pregnancy and STDs. Using methods of birth control other than condoms, such as oral contraceptives, intrauterine devices, and spermicides, does not protect against HIV and other STDs. Questions later in this chapter address the use of spermicides to prevent HIV.

Does cleansing the vagina or anus after sex reduce risk?

No. It is commonly believed that vaginal cleansing, or douching, after sexual intercourse can help prevent pregnancy and STDs, but this is not so. The notion that vaginal cleansing after sex protects against STDs is a myth. In fact, it is likely that vaginal cleansing may actually facilitate HIV infection by washing infected semen deeper into the vagina. The same is true of rinsing the anus after sex.

Condoms

Latex condoms are the only form of birth control that also prevents the spread of STDs, including HIV infection. When used properly, condoms create a barrier between infected body fluids and sex partners. For this reason, condoms are the universal method for preventing HIV infection. Unfortunately, condoms are not always used during sex. The greatest obstacle to using condoms is the belief that condoms interfere with sexual pleasure, stimulation, and spontaneity. A better understanding of condoms and their proper use can help get past negative attitudes, allowing people to protect themselves and their sex partners from HIV infection.

How safe do condoms make sex?

Condoms significantly reduce the risk of HIV infection during sexual intercourse. Research has shown that latex condoms do not allow HIV to pass through. Laboratory studies have tested whether HIV can penetrate latex after it has been stressed in a manner that simulates the friction and wear of sexual intercourse.

In these studies, latex was impermeable for HIV. Just as convincing are studies of couples where one member is HIV positive and the other is not, and they continue to engage in sexual intercourse. Couples who consistently use condoms during intercourse have not experienced much HIV transmission to the uninfected partners, whereas over 80% of couples with one HIV-positive partner who only occasionally use condoms do transmit the virus.

Can HIV pass through condoms?

Studies that involved the use of a variety of methods have shown that HIV does not pass through latex condoms as long as the latex remains intact. In one type of study, the surface of stretched and stressed latex was inspected with high-powered microscopes that did not find openings large enough for HIV to pass through. Other studies have placed the virus, or particles the size of the virus, in latex and tested whether they can pass through the latex under various conditions. These studies have repeatedly shown that unbroken latex condoms do not allow HIV to pass through.

Do lambskin condoms protect against HIV?

No. Lambskin condoms, also called *natural condoms*, are not made of latex. As their name implies, natural-skin condoms are actually made of membranes taken from animals, such as sheep intestine. For many people, natural-skin condoms provide stronger sensations during intercourse because they are porous and allow fluids to cross their membranes. Lambskin condoms prevent pregnancy because they do not allow sperm to pass through. However, because HIV and other viruses are many times smaller than sperm cells, they can easily pass through the pores of natural-skin condoms. Thus, natural-skin condoms offer no protection against HIV and many other STDs.

What are polyurethane condoms?

Polyurethane is a soft and durable material that is thinner than latex and allows for greater transfer of heat during sexual intercourse. Polyurethane condoms are effective at preventing STDs and HIV. For some people, polyurethane condoms may offer greater sexual comfort and increased sensation during vaginal and anal intercourse. Polyurethane condoms are also an option for people who have allergies to latex.

Which condoms offer the best protection?

Latex condoms offer the best protection against HIV infection. Latex condoms have been tested and rated for their strength and durability. As described by *Consumer Reports*, Ramses Extra Ribbed, Sheik Elite, and Lifestyles Vibra-Ribbed have been shown to provide some of the best protection against HIV transmission. *Consumer Reports* provides a detailed account of condom performance that is available by writing to

CU/Reprints, 101 Truman Avenue, Yonkers, NY, 10703-1057.

Is it possible for condoms not to fit?

Latex condoms are made to stretch over the penis to form a snug and comfortably fitting barrier. Condom companies, however, recognize that all men are not built alike and that all condoms do not fit all men. For this reason, condoms are made in regular and larger sizes. Larger size condoms include brand names such as Max and Magnum. It is important, however, that condoms fit properly. Using a condom that is too small can cause unnecessary strain on the latex and increase the chances for breaks or tears. On the other hand, wearing a condom that is too large can allow it to leak from the base or slip off during intercourse.

Are there special condoms made for anal and oral sex?

Most condoms are made for use during vaginal intercourse. There is a greater likelihood that a latex condom will break during anal intercourse than during vaginal intercourse. The anal opening tends to be narrower and less flexible than the vagina. The narrow anal opening increases friction and the strain placed on the latex. Heavier-weight latex condoms are available and add protection during anal intercourse. It is also possible to double up and wear two lubricated latex condoms, one over the other, to increase their strength and reduce the chance of leaks and breaks. With respect to fellatio, the taste of latex, particularly prelubricated latex condoms, can be a real deterrent to using condoms during oral sex. For this reason, there are flavored condoms made specifically for oral sex.

How often do condoms break?

Condom breakage depends on many factors. Condoms are more likely to break when they are old, lubricated with an oil-based product, used during anal intercourse, or used more than once. Research shows that as many as 79% of heterosexual couples who consistently use condoms experience breaks or tears at least once. Overall, between 2% and 5% of condoms break during sexual intercourse. Condoms do not, therefore, entirely remove the risk of HIV transmission, because they can and sometimes do fail. But without question, intercourse with latex condoms is substantially safer than intercourse without condoms.

What is the proper way to use a condom?

Condoms are easy to use, but they are most likely to break when they are worn incorrectly. Proper condom use includes the following:

- Carefully open the package so as not to damage the latex.
- Place a small amount of water-based lubricating jelly in the tip of the condom to increase stimulation and comfort.

- Gently pinch the tip of the condom to assure that there is a reservoir at the tip and that all air bubbles are removed.
- Roll the condom from the tip of the head of the penis all of the way back to the base.
- Remove the condom immediately after intercourse and dispose of it after one use.

When used properly, condoms are the best means of reducing the risks of contracting STDs, including HIV, during sexual intercourse.

Are some condom lubricants better than others?

Yes. Any product made of oil will deteriorate latex and cause the condom to become brittle, thin, and easily damaged. A lubricant must be water-based without any oil, or it will degrade the latex. Water-based lubricants should not be confused with lubricants that are water-soluble. Products that contain oil, such as many hand lotions and body creams, can still be water soluble. See Exhibit 9.3 for commonly used oil-based lubricants that damage latex condoms and water-based lubricants that do not damage latex. Proper lubrication reduces friction and stress on the latex and is necessary for condoms to work properly.

What is the best spermicide for preventing the spread of HIV?

Spermicides are chemicals used as a means of preventing pregnancy. However, some spermicides, particu-

EXHIBIT 9.3. Oil-Based Lubricants That Damage Latex Condoms and Cause Condom Failure, and Water-Based Lubricants That Increase the Effectiveness of Condoms

Oil-based lubricants
- Vaseline petroleum jelly
- Baby oil
- Mineral oil
- Hand lotions with any oil in them, even if water soluble
- Coconut oil
- Cocoa butter

Water-based lubricants
- K-Y Jelly; brand-name medical lubricant
- Spermicide jellies
- Lubricating products made specifically for latex condoms

larly nonoxynol-9, can deactivate HIV in some laboratory experiments. HIV is deactivated as a result of a chemical reaction that interferes with the outer envelope of the virus. Nonoxynol-9 is often contained in foams, jellies, dissolving pellets, films, and creams that are used with barrier methods of birth control. But nonoxynol-9 by itself is not an effective means of preventing the spread of HIV, and some research has suggested that it actually increases risk by causing irritation. Spermicides can be used along with latex condoms, but alone they offer little protection against

HIV. In fact, some people may experience mucous membrane irritation from nonoxynol-9, and this could actually increase the risks for HIV transmission.

How effective is the female condom?

One of the more recent advances in STD prevention is the female condom (brand name Reality Female Condom). The female condom is made of polyurethane, the same plasticlike material that was described earlier for male polyurethane condoms. Polyurethane appears impermeable to HIV. The female condom is a collapsible tube that is open at one end, closed at the other, and conforms to the walls of the vagina. The female condom is inserted with the closed end placed into the vagina. Available research shows that the female condom has a pregnancy failure rate similar to that of male condoms. Research also shows that female condoms do protect against STDs.

Where can a person get free condoms?

Since the beginning of the AIDS epidemic, condoms have become widely available. Latex condoms tend to be inexpensive, costing as little as $5 per dozen, and can be found at pharmacies, convenience stores, and supermarkets. As a part of efforts to stop the spread of HIV, condoms are also often available free from community AIDS organizations, STD clinics, family planning centers, neighborhood clinics, and health departments.

CLEANING NEEDLES

Drugs can be administered in a number of different ways, but it is only when needles are used to inject drugs that a person can become HIV infected. Next to sexual transmission, the sharing of contaminated drug injection equipment most commonly spreads HIV. Just as people can take measures to prevent the sexual spread of HIV, they can take a few simple steps to completely eliminate the risk for HIV infection from needles and other injecting equipment.

Which drugs are the most common carriers of HIV?

It is a myth that drugs themselves cause HIV infection. Research suggests that even drugs that are contaminated with HIV-infected blood do not have active virus that can cause HIV infection. HIV is transmitted by passing the virus from person to person by sharing needles or other injection equipment contaminated with traces of blood. Figure 9.1 shows the typical parts of injection equipment and where HIV can be harbored. It does not matter if a person uses needles to inject heroin, amphetamine, cocaine, steroids, or other drugs; the virus is transmitted through sharing needles and equipment that were previously used by someone with HIV, not the type of drug used.

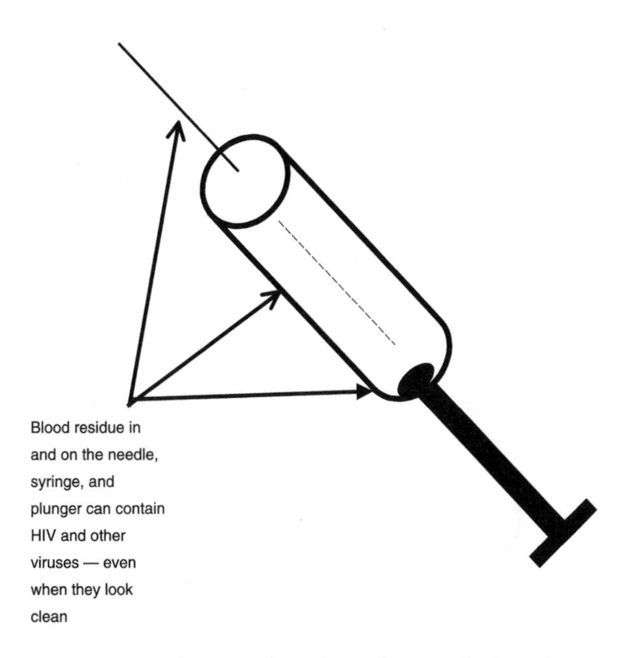

FIGURE 9.1. Typical parts of a syringe that can harbor viruses, including HIV.

What is the best way to clean injection needles?

People who are going to inject drugs can avoid HIV by not sharing needles or other injection equipment with other users. But those who are going to inject with used equipment can reduce their risk of HIV infection by sterilizing the syringe and needles before use. Figure 9.2 shows the proper steps for cleaning injection equipment. It is also important that another person not reuse the rinsing water. Contaminated rinse

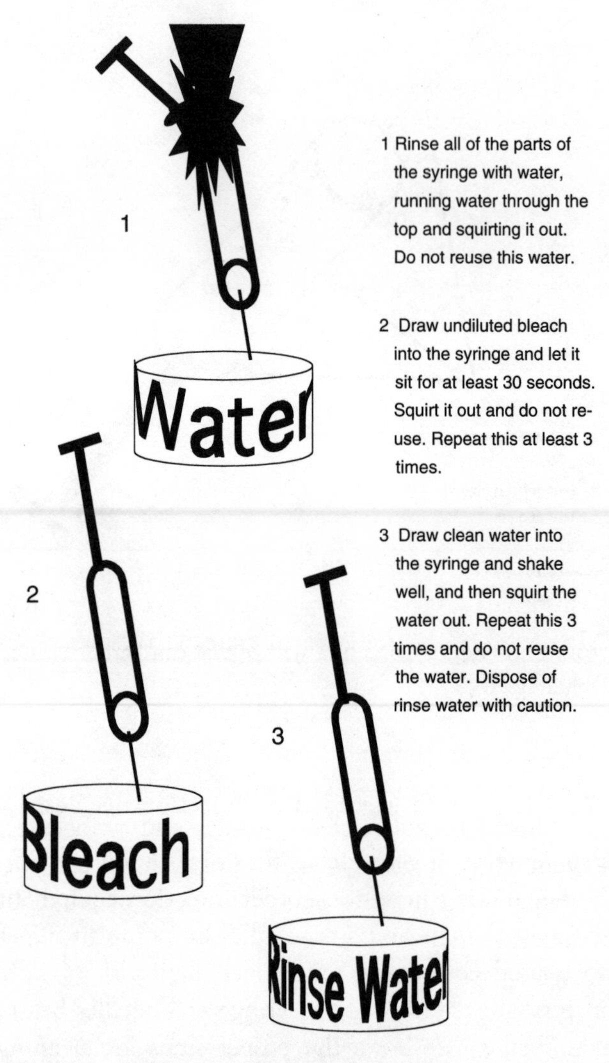

FIGURE 9.2. Proper steps for sterilizing injection needles and syringes.

water can be a source of HIV contamination and should be disposed of down a drain with running water and disinfectant.

Is it OK to use alcohol to clean needles?

No. Alcohol may not inactivate HIV. Cleaning injection equipment in a solution of bleach and water, and following the steps in Figure 9.2, are the best ways to decontaminate injection equipment.

What is *harm reduction*?

Harm reduction is a perspective or philosophy that values the benefits of any reduction in risk, even if the risk is not eliminated. Although the harm reduction perspective can apply to preventing sexually transmitted HIV, it has been discussed most with reference to injection drug use. A harm reduction perspective says that a person who injects drugs should stop. Those who cannot stop should try to get treatment. But if they do not get treatment for their drug addiction, they should be given clean needles and syringes to prevent HIV. If clean needles and syringes are not available to them, they should properly clean their injection equipment and avoid sharing needles and syringes.

What is a needle exchange program?

Needle exchange programs remove the necessity for sharing injection equipment by allowing drug users to swap used for sterile equipment. The first needle exchange programs were established in Europe in the late 1980s. Since then, syringe and needle exchange programs have been established in most major cities, and this has helped prevent the spread of HIV. However, needle exchange is not without controversy. Increasing the availability of injection equipment can be seen as a way of legitimizing and condoning drug abuse. For this reason, communities have had to strike a balance between the public health benefits of preventing HIV infections and the battle against drug abuse.

Do needle exchange programs help prevent the spread of HIV?

Yes. Study after study has demonstrated that access to clean needles and syringes does not promote drug abuse and does prevent HIV infections. In 1997, a panel of leading scientists convened by the National Institutes of Health examined the research on needle exchange programs and concluded the following: An impressive body of evidence suggests powerful effects from needle exchange programs. The number of studies showing beneficial effects of needle exchanges on such behaviors as needle sharing greatly outnumber the studies showing ill effects. There is no longer doubt that these programs work, yet there is striking disjunction between what science dictates and what policy delivers.

Preventing Mother-to-Child HIV Transmission

One of the few great breakthroughs in HIV prevention is the ability to prevent the transmission of HIV from pregnant women to their babies. Pregnant women who know they are HIV positive now have options that, although not 100% effective, do serve to protect their babies.

How can pregnant women protect their children from HIV?

First, pregnant women are advised to get tested for HIV as a part of prenatal care. If a woman tests HIV positive, there are several options available to her; she can take anti-HIV medications during pregnancy, and anti-HIV medications can be administered to the baby. HIV medications are often effective in preventing prenatal HIV transmission and have resulted in drastic reduction in the number of infected babies born to HIV-infected mothers in countries where medications are available.

Can a Caesarian section prevent a woman from infecting her baby?

Research has shown that Caesarian section, or C-section, may help prevent HIV transmission from mother to infant. A C-section involves removing a baby from the uterus by a surgical procedure rather than through vaginal delivery. However, the protection offered by a C-section is considered an additional rather than a substitute safeguard to that offered by the use of anti-HIV medications.

Can an HIV-positive mother breast-feed her baby?

Because HIV is found in breast milk, and because nipples can become irritated and bleed during breast-feeding, HIV-positive mothers are advised not to breast-feed their babies.

Vaccines and Other Prevention Technologies

There are new advances in preventing HIV currently available and others on the horizon. These are just a few questions about such technologies.

What are *universal precautions*?

Universal precautions are steps that should be taken by anyone with the potential to be exposed to blood and other body fluids that may be infected with HIV and other disease-causing agents. These steps generally include

- wearing latex gloves when hands may come in contact with bodily fluids;
- wearing a waterproof apron to protect clothing when there is a possibility that bodily fluids may splash;

- wearing masks or protective eye coverings when there is chance for body substances to splash on the face;
- washing hands frequently, especially scrubbing under the fingernails;
- disposing of uncapped needles and syringes only in specially made, puncture-resistant containers; and
- discarding trash and linens in closed plastic bags.

Is there a vaccine to prevent HIV?

No, not yet. Scientists are working hard to find a safe and effective vaccine for preventing HIV. But the task is far more complicated than that for other vaccines. HIV mutates rapidly so the specific qualities of a vaccine cannot encompass the various strains of HIV. Also, because HIV attacks the immune system, an immune response stimulated by a vaccine is also difficult to achieve. Vaccines are currently under study and being tested on people.

Is there a chemical that can stop HIV?

An area of promising research has been the development of chemicals, or microbicides, that can deactivate HIV on contact. These chemicals may come in jellies or creams and may be placed inside the vagina or anus to stop HIV before it enters the bloodstream. Many studies are testing the safety and effects of microbicides.

What is *postexposure prophylaxis*?

Postexposure prophylaxis, also called *postexposure prevention* or *PEP*, is a procedure that tries to keep a person from getting HIV after possibly having been exposed to the virus. For example, if a person is stuck with a needle that was used on someone who has HIV, it is possible that the person was exposed to the virus. In PEP, the person is immediately, or as close to immediately as possible, given a dose of anti-HIV medications, such as AZT. The person is also kept on the drugs for several weeks while the blood is monitored for evidence of infection. PEP is now used in some cities for people who may be accidentally exposed to HIV, perhaps through a health care occupational accident like a needle stick injury, or when a condom breaks with a known HIV-positive partner, or in cases of rape.

Do anti-HIV medications help prevent the spread of HIV by causing an HIV-positive person to have an undetectable viral load?

No. A person who has HIV and an undetectable viral load can still transmit HIV to others because an undetectable viral load does not mean that HIV is not present. Viral load can change rapidly, so a person who had an undetectable test one day may not be undetectable the next day. Also, the amount of virus necessary to cause HIV infection is unknown, so levels of HIV that are present when a person has an undetectable viral load may be sufficient to cause infection.

Finally, viral load tests are conducted on blood whereas sexual HIV transmission also results from exposure to infected semen and vaginal fluids and there is often no relationship between viral load in blood and viral load in semen or vaginal fluids. Even when people think they have an undetectable viral load, it is likely that their viral load in semen or vaginal fluids is detectable.

Summary

AIDS is completely preventable. People get HIV through direct contact with blood, semen, or vaginal fluids. Avoiding contact with these infectious body fluids assures that a person will not become HIV infected. There is help available for people who want to reduce their risk of HIV infection. Appendix E lists some key contacts including phone numbers and Web sites that offer HIV prevention information and support. Changing behavior, particularly sexual and drug use behavior, is not easy. Support from others including prevention counselors can make a difference in reducing the risk of HIV infection.

Primary Sources for Answers and Suggested Reading

The following books, articles, and reports served as primary sources for most of the answers in this book. They represent the definitive body of current knowledge about AIDS.

Historical Perspectives

Bayer, R., & Oppenheimer, G. (2000). *AIDS doctors: Voices from the epidemic*. New York: Oxford University Press.

A thoughtful account of the history of AIDS as seen through the eyes of doctors who have been there since the beginning. This book offers a unique perspective on AIDS and its impact on doctors and their patients.

Burkett, E. (1995). *The gravest show on earth: America in the age of AIDS*. New York: Houghton-Mifflin.

A historical account of AIDS in America. Describes the social and political context of AIDS in a manner similar to Shilts's *And the Band Played On*.

Gallo, R. C. (1991). *Virus hunting, AIDS, cancer, and the human retrovirus: A story of scientific discovery*. New York: Basic Books.

Dr. Gallo, who is credited with discovering the first human retrovirus, played a major role in discovering HIV. In this book, Dr. Gallo provides his story of how the virus that causes AIDS was discovered.

Hooper, E. (1999). *The river: A journey to the source of HIV and AIDS*. Boston: Back Bay Books.

This book provides detailed analysis of the emergence of AIDS as a global health threat. It also proposes a controversial theory of how AIDS first appeared in Africa, including the potential accidental introduction of HIV through vaccination programs. The book is thought provoking and extremely well-written, and it should be read with a critical eye about the theories it proposes.

Shilts, R. (1987). *And the band played on*. New York: Penguin Books.

Randy Shilts tells the story of how the virus that causes AIDS was discovered, including the political side of science. This book stands alone as personal and historical accounting of the early years of the AIDS epidemic. The movie of the same title is based on the book; it is available from HBO Movies and is also worth seeing.

Biological and Medical Aspects

Aral, S. O., & Holmes, K. K. (1991). Sexually transmitted diseases in the AIDS era. *Scientific American, 264*, 62–69.

Written by two of the foremost leading authorities in the area, this article describes the major sexually transmitted diseases and how they are related to HIV infection.

Baggish, J. (1994). *How your immune system works.* Emeryville, CA: Ziff-Davis.

This book simplifies the human immune system by breaking it down into easy-to-understand parts. It also uses colorful and creative pictures to explain how the immune system works.

Cohen, P. T., Sande, M. A., & Volberding, P. (1999). *The AIDS knowledge base: A textbook on HIV disease from the University of California, San Francisco, and the San Francisco General Hospital.* Philadelphia: Lippincott.

This medical textbook provides a comprehensive overview of all aspects of HIV infection and AIDS.

Hung, F., Conner, R. F., & Villarreal, L. (2000). *AIDS: Science and society (3rd ed.)*. Toronto: Jones & Bartlett.

This useful book provides an overview of HIV/AIDS with excellent sections on modes of HIV transmission and the social aspects of AIDS.

Kloser, P., & Craig, J. M. (1994). *The woman's HIV sourcebook: A guide to better health and well-being*. Dallas, TX: Taylor.

This book addresses specific issues of HIV and AIDS for women. A directory of support services for women and a reference chart for HIV-related conditions in women with HIV also is included.

Marr, L. (1998). *Sexually transmitted diseases: A physician tells you what you need to know*. Baltimore: Johns Hopkins University Press.

This comprehensive book provides a clear and readable account of the transmission and clinical course of sexually transmitted diseases. It is meant to provide patient information and serves as an excellent reference.

Sande, M. A., & Volberding, P. A. (1999). *The medical management of AIDS (6th ed.)*. Philadelphia: W.B. Saunders.

This book is considered by many the most essential textbook on AIDS. The contents describe every aspect of HIV infection and the diseases that bring about a diagnosis of AIDS. Each chapter is written by experts in a specific problem area.

Schoub, B. D. (1993). *AIDS and HIV in perspective*. New York: Cambridge University Press.

This book is a valuable resource for understanding the nature of HIV infection and AIDS. It discusses everything from the virus itself to the diseases that occur after the immune system is damaged. It is very comprehensive and understandable.

Statistical References

Centers for Disease Control and Prevention. (2001). *HIV/AIDS surveillance report*. Atlanta, GA: Author. (Available online at www.cdc.gov)

Published semi-annually, this booklet tracks the course of HIV infections and AIDS cases reported in the United States. It contains many tables and charts that break down the details of the epidemic. This information provides the most accurate accounting of the epidemic available and is free from the CDC.

Mann, J., & Tarantola, D. J. M. (1996). *AIDS in the world II*. New York: Oxford University Press.

Written by international authorities on the state of the AIDS epidemic across the world, this book provides an in-depth look at the extent of the AIDS epidemic on every continent.

UNAIDS. (2001). *Report on the global HIV/AIDS epidemic*. Geneva: WHO. (Available online at www.who.org)

This important document provides a comprehensive overview of the global AIDS crisis. Numerous charts and tables summarize the rates of HIV infections and AIDS cases in all regions of the world. The clearly written text reviews the most important factors that account for the current state of AIDS.

People Living With HIV/AIDS

Callen, M. (1990). *Surviving AIDS*. New York: Harper Perennial.

Michael Callen survived for years after being diagnosed with AIDS. His personal story of this triumph provides inspiration and hope. It is an important account of one man's experience with AIDS.

Kalichman, S. C. (1998). *Understanding AIDS: Advances in treatment and research* (2nd ed.). Washington, DC: American Psychological Association.

This book summarizes and synthesizes the research on mental health and coping among people living with AIDS. Written for mental health professionals, this book is also informative for anyone interested in the biological, medical, and psychological aspects of AIDS.

Legal and Ethical Issues

Gray, J., Lyons, P., & Melton, G. (1995). *Ethical and legal issues in AIDS research.* Baltimore: Johns Hopkins University Press.

This book provides an excellent analysis of the complex ethical and legal issues in AIDS research and care.

Senak, M. A. (1996). *HIV, AIDS, and the law.* New York: Insight Books.

This book offers helpful and practical information for people dealing with the interface of AIDS and the law. Topics include personal wills, child custody, insurance, public assistance, discrimination, and confidentiality.

Terl, A. H. (1992). *AIDS and the law: A basic guide for the non-lawyer.* New York: Hemisphere.

The material in this book is drawn from legal cases involving people with HIV infection and from laws that have emerged to specifically deal with HIV and AIDS. The book addresses issues such as public benefits, criminal law, education, employment, housing, insurance, quarantine, testing, and wills.

Prevention

Cohen, J. (2001). *Shots in the dark: The wayward search for an AIDS vaccine.* New York: Norton.

An excellent accounting of efforts to develop a vaccine to prevent HIV transmission. This book discusses the difficulties researchers face in finding a safe and effective vaccine as well as the social and political aspects of AIDS vaccine research.

Jennings, C. (1993). *Understanding and preventing AIDS: A book for everyone* (7th ed.). Cambridge, MA: Health Alert Press.

This brief booklet provides basic facts about HIV and AIDS. The information is to the point and without much explanation. However, it can be useful as an overview of what HIV is, how it is transmitted, and how it can be prevented.

Kalichman, S. C. (1998). *Preventing AIDS: A sourcebook for behavioral interventions*. Hillsdale, NJ: Erlbaum.

This book reviews the theories and most effective approaches to preventing the sexual transmission of HIV. Grounded in behavioral science research, the book discusses individual, small group, and community level strategies for reducing HIV risk behaviors.

Miller, H. G., Turner, C. F., & Moses, L. E. (1990). *AIDS: The second decade*. Washington, DC: National Academy Press.

Published by the National Research Council's Committee on AIDS research and social science education, this book provides detailed information about the workings of the HIV epidemic and methods that are being used to prevent HIV infection.

NIH Panel. (1997). *National Institutes of Health Consensus Development Statement on Interventions to Prevent HIV Risk Behaviors*. Bethesda, MD: NIH Office of Medical Applications Research.

This report is the result of a thorough analysis of the research on HIV prevention. The summary of research is clear and the report concludes that HIV prevention works, including prevention of sexually and injection-related HIV transmission.

Normand, J., Vlahov, D., & Moses, L. (1995). *Preventing HIV transmission: The role of sterile needles and bleach*. Washington, DC: National Academy Press.

This book provides a review of the scientific research on HIV transmission risks from injection drug use. It also describes prevention programs that work for injection drug users.

APPENDIX A

Glossary

acquired immune deficiency syndrome (AIDS): The final stage of HIV infection, characterized by clinical symptoms of severe *immune deficiency*. Although there are several diagnostic systems, the most widely used is the one provided by the Centers for Disease Control and Prevention, which lists *opportunistic infections* and malignancies that, in the presence of HIV infection, constitute an AIDS diagnosis. In addition, a *T-helper cell count* below 200/mm^3 for people with HIV infection constitutes an AIDS diagnosis.

acute infection: Any infection that begins suddenly, with intense or severe symptoms.

adherence: The degree to which a patient follows drug schedules. A synonym for *compliance*. The act of following a prescribed therapeutic regimen.

AIDS Clinical Trials Group (ACTG): A nationwide consortium of medical centers carrying out clinical trials to study therapies for HIV/AIDS, sponsored by the National Institute of Allergy and Infectious Diseases (NIAID).

AIDS-defining illness: One of the serious illnesses that occurs in HIV-positive individuals and a reason for an AIDS diagnosis according to the definition of AIDS used by the Centers for Disease Control and Prevention. Among these conditions are Pneumocystic carinii pneumonia, AIDS dementia complex, AIDS *wasting syndrome*, *invasive* cervical cancer, *Kaposi's sarcoma*, and CMV *retinitis*.

AIDS-related complex (ARC): A variously defined term with little clinical value used to identify certain HIV-infected individuals prior to an AIDS diagnosis. Compared to earlier in the *epidemic*, the term ARC is used less often today. Instead, physicians chart HIV disease as starting with no apparent *symptoms (asymptomatic)* and progressing to symptoms *(symptomatic)*. Fatigue, night sweats, fever, swollen glands, diarrhea, or unintentional weight loss were previously grouped under the term.

alternative medicine: A catch-all phrase for a long list of treatments of medicinal systems, including traditional systems such as Chinese or Ayurvedic medicine as well as homeopathy, various herbal treatments, and many other miscellaneous treatments that have not been accepted by the mainstream, or Western, medical establishment. Alternative medicine may be referred to as *complementary medicine*.

The designation is not equivalent to *holistic medicine*, which is a more narrow term.

anemia: A decrease in the number of red blood cells or amount of hemoglobin. Commonly called *low blood count*.

anergic: Relating to the *immune system's* inability to produce a marked reaction in response to foreign antigens. For example, HIV-infected individuals who did not react to the tuberculosis skin test even though they have contracted a tuberculosis infection are considered to be anergic.

antibiotic: An agent that kills or inhibits the growth of bacteria, especially a compound similar to those produced by certain fungi for destroying bacteria. An antibiotic is used to combat disease and infection.

antibodies: Molecules in the blood or secretory fluids that tag, destroy, or neutralize bacteria, viruses, or other harmful toxins. They belong to a class of proteins known as *immunoglobulins*, which are produced by B *lymphocytes* in response to antigens.

antiretroviral: Drugs that treat retroviral infection. AZT, ddI, ddC, Crixivan, and Sustiva are examples of antiretrovirals used to treat HIV infection.

apoptosis: A type of cellular suicide triggered by stimulation of particular *receptors* on a cell's surface. It is a metabolic process driven by cellular enzymes in which the cell's chromosomes and then the cell itself breaks down into fragments. In the *immune system*, apoptosis is a process that eliminates unneeded cells. Some researchers believe that accidental apoptosis may be the way that *CD4* cells become depleted in HIV disease, rather than through direct killing by HIV.

assay: A test used to detect the presence and concentration of a drug, virus, or other substance in bodily fluids or tissues.

asymptomatic: Having no *symptoms;* free of sensations of poor health.

attenuated virus: A weakened *virus* with reduced ability to infect or produce disease. Some vaccines are made of attenuated viruses.

bacterium: A microscopic organism composed of a single cell that often causes human disease.

bDNA (branched DNA): A test developed by the Chiron Corporation for measuring the amount of HIV (as well as other viruses) in blood plasma. The test uses a signal amplification technique, which creates a luminescent signal whose brightness depends on the viral RNA present. Test results are calibrated in numbers of virus particle equivalents per milliliter of plasma. bDNA is similar in results, but not in technique, to the *polymerase chain reaction* test, which measures the amount of HIV (as well as other viruses) in blood plasma. The test uses a signal amplification technique, which creates a luminescent signal whose brightness depends on the viral RNA present. Test results are calibrated in numbers of virus particles per mililiter of plasma.

bioavailability: The extent to which an oral medication is absorbed in the digestive tract and reaches the bloodstream.

blinded study: A clinical trial in which participants are unaware whether they are in the experimental or the control group.

B-lymphocytes or B-cells: One of two major classes of *lymphocytes*. During infections, these cells are transformed into plasma cells, which produce large quantities of antibody directed at specific *pathogens*. Although HIV specifically infects cells displaying the *CD4 receptor*, especially T-helper lymphocytes, the disruption of immune function by HIV also affects B lymphocytes; also, B-cell *lymphomas* are common among HIV-positive people.

breakthrough infection: An infection that occurs during the course of a vaccine trial.

Burkitt's lymphoma: A cancerous tumor, frequently involving jaw bones, ovaries, and abdominal *lymph nodes*. The disease is common in Africa and has been associated with *Epstein–Barr virus*.

CD4: A membrane protein or *receptor* of T-helper *lymphocytes*, *monocytes*, *macrophages*, and some other cells; it is the attachment site for HIV.

CD4 count: The most commonly used surrogate marker for assessing the state of the *immune system*. As CD4 cell count declines, the risk of developing *opportunistic infections* increases. The normal range for CD4 cell counts is 500 to 1,500 per cubic millimeter of blood. CD4 count should be rechecked at least every 6 to 12 months if CD4 counts are greater than 500/mm^3. If the count is lower, testing every 3 months is advised.

CD4 percent: The percentage of total *lymphocytes* made up by *CD4* cells. A common measure of immune status is about 40% in healthy individuals and is below 20% in people with AIDS.

CD4/CD8 ratio: The ratio of *CD4* to *CD8* cells. A common measure of *immune system* status that is around 1.5 (to one) in healthy individuals and falls as CD4 counts fall in people with HIV infection.

CD8 (T8): A membrane protein found on the surface of suppressor *T-lymphocytes*.

cell-mediated immunity (CMI): One type of *immune system* response, coordinated by T-helper cells, in which disease is controlled by specific defense cells (cytotoxic *T-lymphocytes*) that kill infected cells.

cellular immunity: Biological defense principally mediated by *lymphocytes* acting directly on invading antigens.

cervical dysplasia: Changes in the lining cells of the cervix that may progress to cancer if not treated in time. Cervical dysplasia is detected through a Pap smear.

chancre: A sore or ulcer. Presence of a chancre on the genitals apparently increases the probability of being infected with HIV.

chemokine: Soluble chemical messengers that attract white blood cells to the site of infection. There are two structural categories of chemokines: alpha (CXC) and beta (cc).

clade: One of the major, largely geographically isolated, HIV subtypes. Classification is based on differences in *envelope* protein. Clade B makes up the overwhelming majority of HIV in North America and Europe.

clotting factors: Substances in the blood that cause the blood to change from a liquid to a coagulate or a solid to stop bleeding.

CMV *retinitis:* CMV infection of the retina. The lesions it causes lead to deterioration in vision and ultimately blindness if untreated.

cofactors: Substances, microorganisms, or characteristics of individuals that influence disease progression.

combination therapy (convergent combination therapies): Combined administration of drugs that are effective at different stages of the HIV viral cycle or that affect different elements of the virus. Combined approaches reduce potential drug *resistance.*

complementary treatments: Unapproved substances or procedures used for therapeutic purposes.

cross-resistance: The phenomenon in which a microbe that has acquired *resistance* to one drug through direct exposure also turns out to have resistance to one or more other drugs to which it has not been exposed. Cross-resistance arises because the mechanism of resistance to several drugs is the same, resulting from identical genetic *mutations*.

cytokines: Chemical messenger proteins released by certain white blood cells, including *macrophages*, *monocytes*, or *lymphocytes*.

cytomegalovirus (CMV): A herpes virus that causes opportunistic diseases in immune-compromised patients. Although CMV can infect most organs of the body, people with AIDS have been most susceptible to CMV *retinitis* and colitis.

cytotoxic T-lymphocyte (CTL): A type of *CD8* or (less often) *CD4 lymphocyte* that kills diseased cells infected by a specific virus or other intracellular microbe. CTLs interact with antigen-bearing MHC class I molecules or infected cells and have a primary role in *cell-mediated immunity*.

encephalopathy: A broad term used to describe metabolic, toxic, malignant, or degenerative diseases of the brain.

endemic: Continuous presence of a disease in a community or among a group of people.

env gene: The gene that encodes spike proteins and glycoproteins of the *envelope* of HIV.

envelope: The outer covering of a virus, sometimes called the *coat*. The HIV envelope is composed of two glycoproteins, *gp41* and *gp120*, which bind to the *CD4* surface molecule.

enzyme: A cellular protein whose shape allows it to hold together several other molecules in close proximity. Enzymes are able in this way to induce chemical reactions in other substances with little expenditure of energy and without being changed themselves. An enzyme is a protein that can cause chemical changes in other substances without undergoing change itself.

enzyme-linked immunosorbent assay (ELISA): The blood test most often used to screen for HIV infection. ELISA detects HIV antibodies, not HIV itself. Because ELISA is sensitive (it has a high false-positive rate), it is confirmed by a more specific test.

epidemic: A disease or condition that affects many people within a population at the same time when ordinarily they are not subject to this condition.

epitope: A unique molecular shape or amino acid sequence carried on a microorganism that triggers a specific antibody or cellular immune response.

Epstein–Barr Virus (EBV): A herpeslike virus that causes mononucleosis, infects the nose and throat, is contagious, lies dormant in the *lymph* glands, and is associated with *Burkitt's lymphoma* and hairy leukoplakia.

erythropoietin: A substance that stimulates bone marrow to produce red blood cells.

gene therapy: Any number of experimental treatments in which cell genes are altered. Some gene therapies attempt to provoke new immune activity; some try to render cells resistant to infection; and some involve the development of enzymes that destroy viral or cancerous genetic material cells.

giant cells: Large multinucleated cells sometimes seen in granulomatous reactions and thought to result from the fusion of *macrophages*.

gp120: A glycoprotein from HIV's *envelope* that binds to *CD4* molecules on cells' outside membrane. Free gp120 in the body may be toxic to cells on its own, causing CD4 depletion in the *immune system* through *apoptosis* and neurological damage leading to AIDS dementia complex.

gp41: A glycoprotein from HIV's outside envelope that joins with gp120 to form the mechanism enabling HIV to latch onto and enter cells.

hepatitis A: A self-limiting virus-induced liver disease. Hepatitis A is acquired through ingesting fecal-contaminated water or food or engaging in sexual practices involving anal contact. Injection drug users who share unclean needles are also at risk.

hepatitis B: A virus-induced liver disease that usually lasts no more than 6 months but becomes chronic and life-threatening in 10% of the cases. The highly contagious hepatitis B virus can be transmitted through sexual contact, contaminated syringes, and blood transfusions.

hepatitis C: A virus-induced liver disease. It appears to be more common among heterosexual people and injection drug users than is *hepatitis* B. It is more likely than hepatitis B to become chronic and lead to liver degeneration (cirrhosis).

heptavax: A vaccine for *hepatitis* B.

herpes simplex virus I (HSV I): Causes cold sores or fever blisters on the mouth or around the eyes and can be transmitted to the genital region; Latent HSV I is reactivated by stress, trauma, other infections, or other causes of *immune suppression*.

herpes simplex virus II (HSV II): Causes painful sores on the anus or genitals; it may lie dormant in nervous tissue and can be reactivated to produce symptoms. It is transmittable to infants during labor and delivery.

herpes varicella zoster virus (HVZ): A virus that causes chicken pox in children; it results in painful blisters on the skin that follow nerve pathways; may reappear in adulthood as herpes zoster causing shingles.

HHV-8 (KSHV, KS herpes virus): A herpes virus thought to trigger the development of *Kaposi's sarcoma* lesions. HHV-8's mode of transmission has not been determined.

highly active antiretroviral therapy (HAART): Aggressive anti-HIV treatment usually including a combination of *protease* and *reverse transcriptase* inhibitors whose purpose is to reduce *viral load* to undetectable levels.

holistic (wholistic) medicine: Various systems of health protection and restoration, both traditional and modern, that are reputedly based on the body's natural healing powers, the various ways the different tissues affect one another, and the influence of the external environment.

human immunodeficiency virus (HIV): The AIDS virus; a *retrovirus* of the lentivirus class; formerly called LAV or HTLV-III. HIV type 1 (HIV-1) is the common cause of HIV disease in the North America; HIV type 2 (HIV-2) is prevalent in some parts of Africa and occasionally occurs in North America and Europe.

human T-cell leukemia virus (HTLV-I): A human *retrovirus* that causes a rare form of leukemia after a long period of *asymptomatic* infection. The virus spreads through sexual contact or the sharing of unclean needles by injection drug users.

immune deficiency: A breakdown or inability of certain parts of the *immune system* to function; a condition that increases susceptibility to certain diseases.

immune reconstitution: The natural or therapy-induced revival of immune function in a body damaged by HIV infection, particularly after initiation of a highly potent antiviral therapy.

immune suppression: A state in which the *immune system* is damaged and does not perform its normal functions; can be induced by drugs or result from diseases.

immune system: The complex body function that recognizes foreign agents or substances, neutralizes them, and recalls the response later when confronted with the same antigen.

immunocompromised: An *immune system* in which the response to infections and tumors is subnormal.

immunodeficiency: A breakdown or an inability of certain parts of the *immune system* to function that renders a person susceptible to certain diseases that he or she ordinarily would not develop.

in vitro (in glass): An artificial environment created outside a living organism (e.g., a test tube or culture plate) used in experimental research to study a disease or process.

in vivo (in life): Studies conducted within a living organism.

incidence: The number of new cases of disease in a defined population during a specified time.

incubation period: The time between infection exposure and the first physical response, such as the production of antibodies.

integrase: The HIV *enzyme* that inserts HIV's genes into a cell's normal DNA. Integrase operates after *reverse transcriptase* has created a DNA version of the RNA form of HIV genes present in virus particles.

interferons: Proteins originally defined by their activity against viral infections. Alpha, beta, and gamma interferons have been investigated as therapy for some opportunistic diseases.

interleukin: One of a large group of glycoproteins that acts as *cytokines*. The interleukins are secreted by and affect many different cells in the *immune system*.

invasive: Disease in which organisms or cancer cells are spreading throughout the body; a medical procedure that involves inserting a device into the body.

isolate: a genetically homogeneous strain of virus that is extracted from a single source with distinguishing characteristics.

Kaposi's sarcoma (KS): A tumor of blood vessel walls, or the lymphatic system; usually appears as pink or purple, painless spots on the skin but may also occur on internal organs.

Langerhans cells: The type of dendritic cell found in the skin.

latency: Latency and *dormancy* (which literally means *sleeping*) mean the same thing: A microbe is in the body but is not actively reproducing, not invading any tissues, and not causing symptoms. Examples of microbes that are latent or dormant in many or most healthy people are *Pneumocystis carinii*, toxoplasma gondii, *herpes simplex virus* (the virus that causes herpes zoster), and *cytomegalovirus*. Once in the body, these microbes remain in the body. They remain latent or dormant until something tilts the balance in the *immune system* and permits them to become active.

lentivirus, slow virus: A virus that produces disease with a greatly delayed onset and protracted course such as HIV.

leukocyte: Any of the various white blood cells, which together make up the *immune system*. Neutrophils, *lymphocytes*, and *monocytes* are all leukocytes.

limit of detection (limit of quantification): The sensitivity of a quantitative diagnostic test, such as the *viral load assay*. The limit of detection is the level below which the test can no longer accurately measure the amount of a substance, such as HIV RNA. If a person has an "undetectable" viral load, it does not mean that HIV is no longer present but rather that the test is not sensitive enough to measure the amount. For *viral load assays, limit of quantification* is becoming the preferred term.

log (logarithm): Formally, the number of times 10 must be multiplied with itself to equal a certain number. For example, 100,000 is log 5 because it is equal to $10 \times 10 \times 10 \times 10 \times 10$. Logs are used to measure changes in *viral load*. For example, a reduction in viral load from 100,000 to 1,000 copies/ml is a two log (or 99%) reduction. Note that half/log change is not a fivefold difference but a change of 3.16-fold (the square root of 10).

long terminal repeat (LTR): The genetic material at each end of the HIV genome. When the HIV genes are integrated into a cell's own genome, the LTR interacts with cellular and viral factors to initiate the transcription of the HIV DNA into an RNA that is packaged in new virus particles. Activation of the LTR is a major step in triggering HIV replication.

long-term nonprogressor: An individual who has been infected with HIV for at least 7 to 12 years (different authors use different time spans) and yet retains a *CD4* cell count within the normal range and shows no evidence of disease progression.

long-term survivor: A looser term than *long-term non-progressor* that indicates any person with any stage of HIV infection, including AIDS, who is stable over a period of years.

lymph: A transparent, slightly yellow fluid that carries *lymphocytes* to and from the lymph nodes and helps to collect foreign microbes. Lymph is derived from tissue fluids. The fluid passes through the lymphatic ducts and then enters the bloodstream.

lymph nodes (glands): Small bean-sized organs of the *immune system*, distributed widely throughout the body. *Lymph* fluid is filtered through *lymph nodes* in which all types of *lymphocytes* take up temporary residence. Antigens that enter the body find their way into lymph or blood and are filtered out by lymph nodes or the spleen.

lymphadenopathy: Swollen, firm, and possibly tender *lymph nodes*; the cause may be an infection or *lymphoma*.

lymphocytes: Several types of white blood cells, including helpers, suppressors, and B- and T-lymphocytes.

lymphoma: A cancer that starts in the *lymph node;* the two major types of lymphoma are Hodgkin's disease and non-Hodgkin's lymphoma (NHL). Lymphoma of the brain is considered an *AIDS-defining illness* unless HIV infection is ruled out.

macrophage: A type of white blood cell that destroys degenerated cells. Macrophages break down antigens.

malaise: A vague feeling of discomfort or uneasiness, often the result of infection or a drug's side effects.

meningitis: An infection of the meninges, the coverings of the brain and spinal cord. Cryptococcus is the most frequent cause of meningitis in HIV infection.

monocyte: A large white blood cell that acts as a scavenger, capable of destroying bacteria or other foreign material; precursor to the *macrophage*.

mutation: Any alteration, loss, gain, or exchange of genetic material within a cell or virus. Mutations are perpetuated in succeeding generations of that cell or virus (or of an entire multicellular organism if the mutated cell is a sperm, egg, or spore). They can occur spontaneously or in response to environmental factors.

naive T-cell: A T-cell arising from the *immune system's* production of fresh cells in the bone marrow. Naive T-cells respond to newly encountered *pathogens* containing antigens the immune system has not processed before. The naive T-cells' activation and proliferation create an acquired immune response to the newly encountered pathogenic agent. After the disease is eradicated, a portion of the T-cell population engendered by the activated naive T-cell constitutes a reservoir of memory cells, which proliferate and respond very quickly to any recurrence of the disease.

natural killer cells (NK cells): Large granular *lymphocytes* that attack and destroy tumor and infected cells; attack without first recognizing specific antigens.

nef: An HIV regulatory protein whose functions are not well understood. HIV without nef appears to have low capacity to infect new cells. Nef also blocks HIV-infected cells from expressing *CD4* and MHC class I molecules on their surfaces, thus limiting the *immune system's* ability to recognize and kill these cells.

neuropathy: An illness involving the nerves. Nerves are responsible for (among other things) the movement of muscles and the sensation of touch, including the sensation of pain. The symptoms of a neuropathy can therefore be weakness of a muscle or pain and tingling. In people with HIV infection, the most frequent symptoms of neuropathy are painful feet and legs.

non-nucleoside reverse transcriptase inhibitor (NNRTI): A member of a class of compounds, including delavirdine and nevirapine, that acts to directly combine with and block the action of HIV's *reverse transcriptase*. In contrast, *nucleoside analogs* block reverse transcriptase by capping the unfinished DNA chain that the *enzyme* is constructing. NNRTIs have suffered from HIV's ability to rapidly mutate and become resistant to their effects.

nucleoside analog: A type of antiviral drug, such as AZT, ddI, ddC, or D4T, whose makeup constitutes a defective version of a natural nucleoside. Nucleoside analogs may take the place of the natural nucleosides, blocking the completion of a viral DNA chain during infection of a new cell by HIV. The HIV *enzyme reverse transcriptase* is more likely to incorporate nucleoside analogs into the DNA it is constructing than is the DNA *polymerase* normally used for DNA creation in cell nuclei.

opportunistic infection: An infection in an immune compromised individual that does not normally occur in healthy people; *pathogens* that cause disease only with immune opportunity.

p24: An HIV-related protein. An indirect measurement of p24 provides an indication of HIV activity; a positive p24 antigen test suggests active HIV replication; p24 antibody levels are usually highest early and late in HIV infection.

palliative: Offering relief of symptoms or comfort without ameliorating the underlying disease process.

pandemic: Denoting a disease affecting the population of an extensive region. HIV disease is a pandemic disease, affecting an extensive area of the world.

papillovirus (HPV): A *virus* that may cause oral, skin, anal, and genital warts or nipplelike growths on the skin.

parasite: An organism that feeds on or lives in a different organism; some parasites cause disease.

parenteral: Involving introduction into the bloodstream.

pathogen: Any *virus*, microorganism, or other substance that causes disease.

pathogenesis: Description of the development of a particular disease, especially the events, reactions, and mechanisms involved at the cellular level.

peripheral neuropathy: A disorder of the nerves, usually involving the extremities. Symptoms include numbness, a tingling or burning sensation, sharp pain, weakness, and abnormal reflexes. In severe cases, paralysis may result.

polymerase: An *enzyme* that promotes synthesis of segments of DNA and RNA.

polymerase chain reaction (PCR): A highly sensitive test that measures the presence or amount of RNA or DNA of a specific organism or *virus* (e.g., HIV or CMV) in the blood or tissue. Unlike the standard blood test for HIV infection that detects antibodies to HIV, the PCR detects HIV itself. PCR tests are being used to gauge HIV disease progression and the effect of particular treatments on HIV infection.

postexposure prophylaxis (PEP): Drug treatment to prevent disease in an individual after exposure to an infectious organism. For example, guidelines have been established for the treatment of health care providers who have been exposed to HIV through needle sticks.

primary HIV infection: The flulike *syndrome* that occurs immediately after a person contracts HIV. This initial infection precedes *seroconversion* and is characterized by fever, sore throat, headache, skin rash, and swollen glands. Also called *acute infection*.

prophylaxis: Prevention; a treatment intended to preserve health.

protease: An *enzyme* that triggers the breakdown of proteins. HIV's protease enzyme breaks apart long strands of viral protein into separate proteins constituting the viral core and the enzymes it contains. HIV protease acts as new virus particles are budding off a cell membrane.

protease inhibitors: Compounds that block the ability of HIV to produce the *enzyme protease*, an essential enzyme for HIV replication.

provirus: The form of a *virus* in which its genetic material is incorporated into the host cell's genetic material.

receptor: A cell's surface molecule which binds specifically to other particular extracellular molecules.

resistance (to a drug): The ability of an organism, a microorganism, or a virus to lose its sensitivity to a drug. For example, after long-term use of AZT, HIV can develop strains of virus in the body that are no longer suppressed by the drug and therefore are said to be resistant to AZT. Resistance is thought to result from a genetic *mutation*. In HIV, such mutations can change the structure of viral enzymes and proteins so that an antiviral drug can no longer bind with them as well as it used to. Resistance detected by searching a *pathogen's* genetic makeup for mutations thought to confer lower susceptibility is called *genotypic resistance*. Resistance found by successfully growing laboratory cultures of the pathogen in the presence of a drug is called *phenotypic resistance*. High-level resistance reduces a drug's virus-suppressing activity hundreds of times; low-level resistance represents a lesser reduction in drug effectiveness. Depending on the *toxicity* of the drug, low-level resistance may be overcome by using higher doses of the drug in question.

retinitis: Inflammation of the retina. Retinitis can diminish vision, contract visual fields, and increase light sensitivity. *Cytomegalovirus* infection is a cause in immune suppressed persons.

retrovirus: A class of RNA *viruses* with a complex life cycle that includes an obligatory DNA intermediate and reverse transcription from RNA to DNA and is almost impossible for the body to eliminate. A retrovirus takes over cells in the body and makes them into factories that produce other infected cells, each with a slightly different retrovirus.

rev: A regulatory protein produced by HIV within infected cells. Rev helps transport HIV RNA sequences (messenger RNA) out from the nucleus into the cell's cytoplasm, where it directs construction of proteins for new virus particles.

reverse transcriptase (RT): A viral *enzyme* that transcribes viral RNA into DNA so that genetic material of the virus can be integrated into genetic material of the T-cell helper and other host cells. Many antivirals inhibit the action of this enzyme, including AZT, ddI, and ddC.

ribonucleic acid (RNA): A complex nucleic acid responsible for translating genetic information from DNA and transferring it to the cells' protein-making machinery.

seroconversion: When people exposed to an infectious disease develop *antibodies* to that disease-causing agent; people seroconvert from antibody negative to antibody positive.

serologic test: Tests performed on the clear, liquid portion of blood (serum); often refers to tests that determine the presence of *antibodies* to antigens. *ELISA* and *Western blot* are two types of antibody tests.

serostatus: The condition of having or not having detectable *antibodies* to a microbe in the blood as a result of infection. One may have either a positive or negative serostatus.

simian immunodeficiency virus (SIV): A *retrovirus* that causes *immune deficiency* in some species of monkeys. This virus does not infect humans.

stem cell: A cell in bone marrow that can grow into many types of *immune system* cells.

suppressor T cells (T8, CD8): Subset of T cells that halt antibody production and other immune responses.

surrogate marker: A laboratory measurement or physical sign that does not directly show how patients feel, but rather predicts the likely effect of a medication on their future disease status. *CD4* cell count is an example of a surrogate marker in HIV infection.

symptom: Feelings or sensations that may indicate disease that are not observable but are reported; examples include headache, nausea, and pain.

symptomatic: A person who doesn't feel well and has medical problems that can be observed or measured.

syncytium ("giant cell"): A dysfunctional multicellular clump formed by cell-to-cell fusion.

syndrome: A group of *symptoms* and diseases that together are characteristic of a specific condition.

synergy (adj.: synergistic): The interaction of two or more treatments such that their combined effect is greater than the sum of the individual effects observed when each treatment is administered alone.

tat: An HIV protein that helps produce new complete HIV RNA genomes, and ultimately new virus, from the HIV proviral DNA template present in infected cells. Tat may also be involved in (a) the reactivation of other latent viruses in people with AIDS, (b) the development of AIDS-related *Kaposi's sarcoma* by stimulating the formation of new blood vessels, and (c) the triggering of anery and *apoptosis* in *CD4* cells.

tat inhibitors: Experimental drugs that block HIV's *tat* gene.

T-helper cell count: The most commonly used laboratory marker for estimating level of immune dysfunction; also known as *lymphocyte count* or *CD4 count*; a measurement of number of T-helper cells per unit of blood.

thymus: The central lymphoid organ that is present in the thorax and controls the ontogeny of *T-lymphocytes*.

T-lymphocytes or T-cells: The class of *lymphocytes* derived from the *thymus* and involved in cell-mediated immune responses.

TMP/SMX (Bactrim, Septra): Used for prevention or treatment of PCP.

toxicity: The harmful side effects of a given drug.

treatment-naive: Refers to patients with no history of previous treatment for a particular condition.

T-suppressor lymphocytes (T-8 cells): A group of *T-lymphocytes* that regulates the antibody production of B lymphocytes.

vaccination: Immunization with antigens administered for the prevention of infectious diseases.

viral load: The amount of HIV RNA per unit of blood plasma. An indicator of virus concentration and reproduction rate, HIV viral load is increasingly used as a predictor of disease progression. It is measured by PCR and *bDNA* tests and is expressed in numbers of copies of or equivalents to the HIV RNA genome per milliliter of plasma. (Note that there are two RNA copies per HIV *virion*.)

viremia: The presence of virus in the blood or blood plasma. Plasma viremia is a quantitative measurement of HIV levels similar to *viral load* but is accomplished by seeing how much of a patient's plasma is required to start an HIV infection in a laboratory cell culture.

virion: A virus particle existing freely outside a host cell.

virus: A group of infectious agents characterized by their inability to reproduce outside of a living host cell; may subvert the host cell's normal functions, causing the cell to behave in a manner determined by the virus.

wasting syndrome: Progressive, involuntary weight loss associated with advanced HIV infection.

Western blot: A test for detecting specific *antibodies* to a particular *pathogen*. In testing for antibodies to HIV, a Western blot test confirms a positive *ELISA* screening blood test.

APPENDIX B

Answer Key to HIV/AIDS Knowledge Questionnaire

It is expected that everyone will miss some questions on this test. Each answer is followed by the page number in the text where you can learn more about the area addressed in each question.

1.	False	(p. 19)
2.	False	(p. 202)
3.	False	(p. 158)
4.	True	(p. 158)
5.	True	(p. 103)
6.	True	(p. 85)
7.	False	(p. 166)
8.	False	(p. 19)
9.	False	(p. 165)
10.	False	(p. 162)
11.	True	(p. 261)
12.	True	(p. 154)

13. True (p. 116)
14. True (p. 106)
15. False (p. 248)
16. True (p. 90)
17. False (p. 249)
18. True (p. 92)
19. False (p. 243)
20. False (p. 106)
21. True (p. 250)
22. False (p. 249)
23. False (p. 249)
24. True (p. 78)
25. True (p. 57)
26. False (p. 36)
27. False (p. 48)
28. True (p. 57)
29. False (p. 265)
30. True (p. 199)
31. True (p. 169)
32. False (p. 193)
33. False (p. 96)
34. False (p. 88)
35. True (p. 109)
36. True (p. 106)
37. False (p. 251)
38. False (p. 62)
39. False (p. 100)
40. True (p. 48)
41. False (p. 141)
42. False (p. 94)

43. False	(p. 57)
44. True	(p. 257)
45. False	(p. 251)
46. False	(p. 265)
47. True	(p. 109)
48. False	(p. 177)
49. False	(p. 158)
50. False	(p. 33)
51. True	(p. 30)
52. True	(p. 135)
53. True	(p. 263)
54. False	(p. 88)
55. True	(p. 97)
56. False	(p. 194)
57. False	(p. 255)
58. False	(p. 259)
59. True	(p. 92)
60. True	(p. 103)
61. False	(p. 249)
62. False	(p. 243)

APPENDIX C

Symptoms of Sexually Transmitted Diseases

Bacteria, viruses, and other parasites that infect a person through sexual contact cause sexually transmitted diseases (STDs). Unless treated, sexually transmitted infections can cause damage to body organs, result in infertility, and even be fatal. Symptoms of STDs require examination by trained health care providers.

Bacterial Infections

Syphilis

The corkscrew-shaped bacterium *Treponema palladium* causes *syphilis*, a serious infection that originates from contact with infected mucous membranes. Syphilis starts out as an infection at the site of transmission, usually the genitals. Early symptoms include an open sore (*chancre*) where the bacteria entered the body, skin rash, fever, headache, and muscle aches. If treated with antibiotics, however, syphilis is completely curable in its early stages. If left untreated, it can progress to an untreatable and lethal infection.

Gonorrhea

Gonorrhea is caused by the round-shaped bacterium *Neisseria gonorrhea*. Like syphilis, gonorrhea is transmitted from person to person during contact with infected mucous membranes. Gonorrhea in men causes urinary tract infection; symptoms include painful urination and a discharge from the penis. In women, gonorrhea usually infects the cervix, causing a discharge that can easily go unnoticed in its early stages. If undetected, gonorrhea can progress to an inflammatory infection that spreads throughout the woman's pelvic region. Gonorrhea can also infect the throat and rectum. When diagnosed in its early stages, gonorrhea is usually cured with antibiotics.

Chlamydia Trachomatis

Chlamydia trachomatis is a bacterium that is sexually transmitted and infects the urethra in men and the cervix in women. Like gonorrhea, men more readily notice the symptoms of chlamydia infection than women, making the risk for a worsening infection greater for women. When diagnosed, antibiotics treat chlamydia infections.

Viral Infections

Herpes Simplex Virus Type-2

Herpes simplex virus type-2 belongs to the common family of herpes viruses. Typically, this is the virus that causes genital herpes. However, herpes simplex virus type-1, the virus that causes cold sores, can also be transmitted to the genitals. Herpes simplex virus causes painful blisters that erupt in the area where contact with the virus took place. Blisters occur periodically, usually triggered by stress of another illness or other factors that suppress the immune system's control of the infection. Outbreaks of herpes blisters cause itching and burning that lasts about 2 to 3 weeks and then completely clears up, after which the virus lays dormant for periods of time. Herpes simplex viruses are transmitted during contact between mucous membranes, such as oral, vaginal, or anal sex,when one person is having an outbreak. A herpes outbreak in the vagina during childbirth can transmit the virus to the skin of the baby, causing an infection that can be deadly. Like many viral infections, herpes can be treated to relieve some of the symptoms, but it cannot be cured.

Hepatitis B

Hepatitis B is one of a few viruses to cause a serious infection of the liver. Unlike other hepatitis viruses, however, hepatitis B virus is sexually transmitted. Hepatitis can ultimately cause severe liver damage.

APPENDIX D

AIDS-Defining Opportunistic Illnesses

Following is a brief description of the illnesses included in the 1993 AIDS diagnosis. For AIDS to be diagnosed, the disease must occur in the presence of HIV infection.

Pneumocystis carinii pneumonia (PCP). PCP is the most frequently occurring AIDS-defining condition in people with HIV infection in the United States. It exists in the environment, and it is believed that everybody inhales it at some point. However, it only becomes a health threat when the immune system has been severely damaged, particularly when T-helper lymphocyte cell counts fall below 200. PCP is associated with the following symptoms: chest pain, chronic fever, fatigue, weight loss, and a dry cough with shortness of breath.

Kaposi's sarcoma. Although rare before the HIV epidemic, Kaposi's sarcoma has become the most common malignancy among people with AIDS, with the majority of cases occurring among men who sexually contracted HIV from other men. This is because a virus that is sexually transmitted causes Kaposi's sarcoma. Kaposi's sarcoma is usually a mass on the skin, mucous membranes, or internal organs. The first sign of the disease consists of a dark red to violet-colored area in people with light skin, and black or brown in people with dark skin. Kaposi's sarcoma also carries a psychological burden because the symptoms are disfiguring and their appearance will frequently mark a person as being seriously ill and can often lead to diagnosing a person with AIDS.

It is common for Kaposi's sarcoma to appear on the head, face, and neck. Like most types of cancer, Kaposi's sarcoma can spread. Lesions on the skin look like bruises and can appear anywhere on the body. The lesions can be very small or quite large. Kaposi's sarcoma can become life-threatening when it invades the intestinal system and other internal organs. There are medications, however, to control the progression of the disease.

HIV-related wasting. Although several diseases affect the digestive system that cause chronic weight loss, HIV itself can directly cause these symptoms. HIV wasting usually involves long bouts of chronic diarrhea, fever, weight loss, fatigue, lethargy, and physical weakness.

HIV-related neurological disease. Disturbances in thinking and behavior can occur with AIDS, especially at the later stages. HIV-related neurological disease can include difficulty maintaining concentration, memory problems, and motor disturbances, including slowing of arm, leg, and eye movements. In severe cases, the ability to work, care for oneself, and have relationships becomes impaired.

Cytomegalovirus (CMV). CMV is a type of herpes virus and is a very common cause of disease in HIV infection. This infection can cause colitis, inflammation of the esophagus, pneumonia, and liver disease. However, CMV is most infamous for causing loss of vision from retinitis (infection of the retinas).

Herpes simplex virus infection. People with HIV infection who are also infected with herpes simplex virus can have long bouts of small, painful, erupting blisters. Although herpes blisters normally heal within 3 to 4 weeks, people with AIDS may have prolonged outbreaks that last months.

Epstein-Barr virus and hairy leukoplakia. Epstein-Barr virus causes infectious mononucleosis with symptoms of fatigue and swollen lymph glands. For people with HIV infection, Epstein-Barr virus is also related to hairy leukoplakia, which causes white lesions on the tongue and inside the mouth.

Progressive multifocal leukoencephalopathy (PML). Caused by a human papovavirus, PML causes progressive and fatal brain damage. Symptoms include changes in mental status, memory, and language; headache; seizures; and loss of movement.

Candidiasis. Candida is a fungus that normally exists in the mouth and esophagus of healthy people.

With immune suppression, such as the loss of T-helper cells, however, candida can become an active disease. Oral infection with candidiasis is commonly called *thrush*, usually forming removable white plaques or small red areas on the surface of the tongue and inside the mouth. For an AIDS diagnosis, candidiasis must involve the esophagus, lungs, or trachea. Infection can also occur in the digestive system and vagina.

Coccidioidomycosis. An infection that occurs after fungus particles are inhaled into the lungs, coccidioidomycosis is among the least common AIDS illnesses in North America. Risk for coccidioidomycosis is greatest in areas where the fungus is abundant, including the southwestern United States. Coccidioidomycosis can remain in the lungs or can be spread to other organs of the body. However, coccidioidomycosis is diagnosed as AIDS only when it spreads beyond the lungs.

Cryptococcoses. Cryptococcal infection tends to occur with very severe immune suppression. Although the disease often affects the lungs, the most common form of infection is cryptococcal meningitis, infection of the outer coverings of the brain and spinal cord. The symptoms of meningitis include headache, stiff neck, nausea, vomiting, sensitivity to light, malaise, and possibly seizures.

Histoplasmosis. Like other fungal infections, histoplasmosis gets into the body by the inhalation of fungus particles in places where the fungus grows, with infection possibly moving to other parts of the body. Symptoms of this infection include fever, skin rashes, anemia, and swollen lymph nodes.

Cryptosporidiosis. Infection with cryptosporidiosis occurs after spores are either inhaled or ingested. Cryptosporidia infects the digestive system, usually the small intestine, and causes chronic, disabling, and even deadly diarrhea. Outbreaks in cities where drinking water has been contaminated by cryptosporidium have caused several deaths among people with suppressed immune systems, particularly infants, the elderly population, people undergoing cancer chemotherapy, and people with AIDS.

Isosporiasis. Isosporiasis has been a rare infection in people with AIDS in the United States. Like cryptosporidia this infection strikes the gastrointestinal tract, causing diarrhea, cramping, and weight loss. However, unlike other protozoan infections, effective treatments are available for isosporiasis.

Toxoplasmosis. *Toxoplasma gondii* is the cause of toxoplasmosis, the most common infection of the human brain. People usually come in contact with *Toxoplasma gondii* through contact with cat feces; house cats are common carriers of *Toxoplasma gondii*. The disease can cause a mixture of neurological symptoms, including disturbed thoughts, lethargy, confusion, memory loss, language problems, and movement disorders.

Invasive cervical cancer. Cervical cancer in women with HIV infection comes from increased immune suppression. Invasive cervical cancer was first included in the 1993 AIDS diagnosis.

HIV-related lymphomas. Unlike other lymphomas, those related to HIV infection tend to progress rapidly and have a rather grim prognosis. Although most non-HIV infected lymphomas involve disease contained inside of the lymph nodes, HIV lymphomas are apt to spread throughout the body. Most commonly, HIV-related lymphomas spread to the brain, posing a serious threat, one that is rare with non-HIV lymphomas.

Mycobacterium diseases. Mycobacterial infections include mycobacterium tuberculosis (TB), Mycobacterium Avium Complex (MAC), and other disseminated mycobacteria. TB can spread to a number of organ systems. The course of TB in people with AIDS is usually rapid and severe. Symptoms may include fever, night sweats, fatigue, malaise, and weight loss. Symptoms also usually include chest pain and a nagging cough that produces a lot of mucus.

MAC also is common to HIV infection. The disease is contracted through contaminated soil, food, water, and air-water droplets. Symptoms of MAC infection include fever, weight loss, malaise, severe anemia, serious loss of appetite, and numerous digestive system problems, such as chronic diarrhea, abdominal pain, and malabsorption.

Recurrent bacterial pneumonia. Pneumonia caused by any one of several different bacteria is frequently seen in people with HIV infection. Bacterial pneumonia typically comes on quickly and lasts several days.

Pneumonia in HIV infection is similar to most cases of pneumonia and includes fever, cough, labored or difficult breathing, and chest pain. However, symptoms of pneumonia in people with HIV infection persist for long periods of time.

APPENDIX E

Directory of Local and National Resources for HIV/AIDS

Toll Free Telephone Information Directory

The CDC National AIDS Hotline is operated 24 hours a day, 7 days a week. The hotline serves more than 1 million people each year. AIDS information experts are available to answer questions, provide referral sources, and send free information brochures by e-mail and postal mail. The National AIDS Hotline also can provide phone numbers to local AIDS organizations, HIV testing centers, local hotlines, and health departments.

CDC National AIDS Hotline	800-342-2437
CDC National AIDS Hotline TTY Service	800-243-7889
CDC National AIDS Hotline Spanish Service	800-344-7432
CDC National STD Hotline	800-227-8922

State AIDS Hotlines

Note that the numbers that follow are subject to change. If the number listed here is not current, you can obtain an updated number from the CDC National AIDS Hotline listed previously.

Alabama	800-228-0469
Alaska	800-478-2437
	907-276-4880
Arkansas	800-342-2437
Arizona	800-342-2437
California	800-367-AIDS
San Francisco	415-863-2437
TDD	888-225-AIDS
Colorado	800-252-2437
Denver	303-782-5186
Connecticut	800-381-2437
Delaware	800-422-0429
District of Columbia	202-332-2437
Metro DC & Virginia	800-322-7432
Florida (English)	800-352-AIDS
Haitian Creole	800-243-7101
Spanish	800-545-SIDA
TTY	888-503-7118
Georgia	800-551-2728
	404-876-9944
Hawaii	800-321-1555
	808-922-1313
Idaho	800-926-2588

Illinois	800-243-2437
TTY/TDD	800-782-0423
Indiana	800-848-2437
TTY/TDD	800-972-1846
Iowa	800-445-2437
Louisiana	800-992-4379
	504-944-2437
TDD	504-944-2492
Maine	800-851-2437
	800-775-1267
Maryland (bilingual)	800-638-6252
Metro DC & Virginia	800-322-7432
Massachusetts	800-235-2331
	617-536-7733
TTY/TDD	617-437-1672
Michigan	800-872-2437
TTY/TDD	800-332-0849
Spanish	800-826-SIDA
Teen line	800-750-TEEN
Minnesota	800-248-2437
	612-373-2437
Mississippi	800-826-2961
Missouri	800-533-2437
Montana	800-233-6668
Nebraska	800-782-2437
Nevada	800-842-2437
New Hampshire	800-752-2437
New Jersey	800-624-2377
TTY/TDD	201-926-8008
New Mexico	800-545-2437

New York	800-872-2777
	800-541-2437
Spanish	800-233-SIDA
Deaf and hearing impaired	800-369-2437 TDD
New York City	800-TALK-HIV
North Carolina	800-342-2437
North Dakota	800-782-2437
	701-328-2378
Ohio	800-332-2437
TTY/TDD	800-332-3889
Oklahoma	800-535-2437
Oregon	800-777-2437
Voice & TTY	503-223-2437
Pennsylvania	800-662-6080
Puerto Rico	800-981-5721
	809-765-1010
Rhode Island	800-726-3010
South Carolina	800-322-2437
South Dakota	800-592-1861
Tennessee	800-525-AIDS
Texas	800-299-2437
Utah	800-366-2437
	801-487-2100
Vermont	800-882-2437
Virgin Islands	809-773-2437
Virginia	800-533-4148
Spanish	800-322-7432
Washington	800-272-2437
West Virginia	800-642-8244

Wisconsin	800-334-2437
	414-273-2437
Wyoming	800-327-3577

AIDS Information Online: Internet Directory

Biological and Medical Aspects of AIDS

AIDS Pathology
http://www-medlib.med.utah.edu/WebPath/TUTORIAL/AIDS/AIDS.html#10
Harvard AIDS Institute Basic Science links
http://www.hsph.harvard.edu/hai/resources/basic/index.html
JAMA HIV/AIDS Info Center
http://www.ama-assn.org/special/hiv/
NOVA Online—Surviving AIDS
http://www.pbs.org/wgbh/nova/aids/
Understanding the Immune System
http://rex.nci.nih.gov/PATIENTS/INFO_TEACHER/bookshelf/NIH_immune/index.html

Treatments and Clinical Trials

Adult AIDS Clinical Trials Group (AACTG)
http://aactg.s-3.com/
American Foundation for AIDS Research (AmFAR)
http://www.amfar.org
AIDS Treatment News—Online
http://www.aids.org/immunet/atn.nsf/homepage

Being Alive Newsletter
http://www.beingalivela.org/newsletter.html
BETA: Bulletin of Experimental Treatments for AIDS
http://www.sfaf.org/beta/
Body Positive
http://www.thebody.com/bp/bpix.html#magazine
Canadian HIV Trials Network
http://www.hivnet.ubc.ca/ctn.html
Clinical Trials.gov
http://www.clinicaltrials.gov/
Division of Acquired Immunodeficiency Syndrome (DAIDS), National Institute of Allergy & Infectious Diseases (NIAID), National Institutes of Health (NIH)
http://www.niaid.nih.gov/daids/default.htm.
Forum for Collaborative HIV Research
http://www.hivforum.org/
HIV Medication Guide
http://www.jag.on.ca/asp_bin/Main.asp
National Institutes of Health Clinical Trials Database
http://clinicalstudies.info.nih.gov/
Office of AIDS Research
http://www.nih.gov/od/oar/
Pediatric AIDS Clinical Trials Group
http://pactg.s-3.com/
Positively Aware
http://www.tpan.com/

Alternative Therapies

Alternative Medicine Homepage
 http://www.pitt.edu/~cbw/altm.html
Alternative Medicine Review
 http://www.thorne.com/altmedrev/index.html
Being Alive Web Site
 http://www.mbay.net/~bngalive/index.html
National Institutes of Health, National Center for Complementary and Alternative Therapies
 http://nccam.nih.gov

Research and Reference

AIDS Education Global Information Service Database
 http://www.aegis.org/
AIDS Resource List
 http://www.specialweb.com/aids
AIDS-HIV Book Store
 http://www.wellnessbooks.com/IDS/
AIDS-HIV Resource Guide
 http://www.healingwell.com/AIDS/
Association of Nurses in AIDS Care (USA)
 http://www.anacnet.org/
12th National HIV/AIDS Update Conference
 http://www.nauc.org/
Harvard AIDS Institute
 http://www..edu/hai/home.html
HIVInsite
 http://hivinsite.ucsf.edu/

Lancet
http://www.thelancet.com/
Medscape
http://hiv.medscape.com
New Mexico AIDS InfoNet
http://www.aidsinfonet.org
Project Inform
http://www.projinf.org
Retrovirus & Opportunistic Infections Conferences
http://www.retroconference.org/
XIII International Conference Abstracts
http://www.iac2000.org/
What About AIDS
http://www.nyhallsci.org/whataboutaids/main.html

Prevention

AETC National Resource Center
http://www.aids-ed.org
Center for AIDS Prevention Studies (CAPS) AIDS Prevention Fact Sheets
http://www.caps.ucsf.edu/FSindex.html
CDC Division of HIV/AIDS Prevention (DHAP)
http://www.cdc.gov/hiv/dhap.htm
Coalition for Positive Sexuality
http://www.positive.org/Home/index.html
HIV InSite Prevention and Education
http://hivinsite.ucsf.edu/InSite.jsp?page+Prevention
HIV Stops With Me
http://www.hivstopswithme.org/2001/index.html

North American Syringe Exchange Network
http://www.nasen.org/
Red Cross HIV/AIDS Education
http://www.redcross.org/services/hss/hivaids/
Rural Center for AIDS/STD Prevention
http://www.indiana.edu/~aids/
San Francisco AIDS Foundation
http://www.sfaf.org/prevention/
Stop AIDS Project
http://www.stopaids.org/

Advocacy

ACT UP-New York
http://www.actupny.org/
African American AIDS Policy and Training Institute
http://www.BlackAIDS.org
AIDS Action Council
http://www.aidsaction.org/
AIDS Drug Assistance Program (ADAP) Working Group
http://www.aidsinfonyc.org/awg/index.html
AIDS Empowerment and Treatment International
http://www.aidseti.org/
AIDS/HIV Law and Policy Resource
http://www.critpath.org/aidslaw/index.html#resource
National Association of People With AIDS
http://www.napwa.org/
National Minority AIDS Council
http://www.nmac.org

Online Glossaries

AIDS Education Global Information Service Online Glossary
http://www.aegis.com/ni/topics/glossary/
HIV/AIDS Treatment Information Service
http://glossary.hivatis.org/index.asp
San Francisco AIDS Foundation Glossary
http://www.sfaf.org/treatment/glossary/

Government Web Sites

Centers for Disease Control, Division of HIV/AIDS Prevention (DHAP)
http://www.cdc.gov/hiv/dhap.htm
Food & Drug Administration HIV/AIDS Page
http://www.fda.gov/oashi/aids/hiv.html
Health Resources and Services Administration (HRSA) HIV/AIDS Services
http://hab.hrsa.gov
National Institutes of Health Office of AIDS Research
http://www.nih.gov/od/oar/
World Health Organization
http://www.who.org

Index

About the Author

Seth C. Kalichman received his PhD in clinical-community psychology from the University of South Carolina in 1990. He is a professor in the Psychology Department at the University of Connecticut and has previously been on the faculties of Loyola University of Chicago, Georgia State University, and the Medical College of Wisconsin. His research focuses on AIDS prevention, treatment, and care. He conducts studies to identify better ways to prevent the spread of HIV and to improve the health and quality of life of those already infected with HIV. His research is supported by the National Institute of Mental Health. Dr. Kalichman also serves on several advisory boards, editorial boards, and National Institute of Health grant review committees. He was the 1997 recipient of the Distinguished Scientific Award for Early Career Contribution to Psychology in Health awarded by the American Psychological Association (APA). He is an associate editor of the journal *Health Psychology* and the author of three other books, including *Understanding AIDS* (APA, 1996).